Complementary Medicine

New Approaches to Good Practice

The British Medical Association (BMA) is a professional organization representing all doctors in the UK. It was established in 1832 'to promote the medical and allied sciences, and to maintain the honour and interests of the medical profession'. The BMA Board of Science and Education supports this aim by providing an interface between the profession, the government, and the public, and by undertaking research studies on behalf of the Association. Through the publication of policy statements the Board of Science has led the debate on key public health issues.

The overriding objective of the Board of Science is to contribute to the development of better public health policies that affect the community, the state, and the medical profession. In order to do this, investigations need to be carried out by the Board on the impact of various policies and activities on the public health. The Board appoints working parties, combining medical and other specialist expertise, to carry out research on a variety of important issues. The Board has produced a large number of publications over recent years reflecting current concerns in the public health arena, such as alcohol and tobacco abuse, AIDS, nutrition, infection control, hazardous waste, and chemical pesticides.

The BMA Board of Science and Education investigates issues which may affect the health of the community and the health care which it receives. In the UK, health care is provided by a range of services and people, from counsellors and chiropodists to doctors and nurses. There are increasing numbers of non-conventional therapists who also offer different forms of treatment for the individual. This book studies complementary medicine as a public-health issue, examining measures to safeguard consumers of such therapies from possible harm. In this way, the report extends the work of the Board in promoting the safety and good health of the nation.

A publication from the BMA Scientific Division

Chairman, Board of Science and Education	Professor Jack Howell
Project Director	Dr Fleur Fisher
Editor	David Morgan
Written by	Tara Lamont
Contributor	Simon Fielding
Editorial Secretariat	Sallie Robins
Design	Hilary Glanville

Complementary Medicine

New Approaches to Good Practice

British Medical Association

Oxford   New York

OXFORD UNIVERSITY PRESS

1993

Oxford University Press, Walton Street, Oxford OX2 6DP

Oxford New York Toronto
Delhi Bombay Calcutta Madras Karachi
Kuala Lumpur Singapore Hong Kong Tokyo
Nairobi Dar es Salaam Cape Town
Melbourne Auckland Madrid

and associated companies in
Berlin Ibadan

Oxford is a trade mark of Oxford University Press

© British Medical Association 1993

First published 1993 as an Oxford University Press paperback

British Library Cataloguing in Publication Data
Data available

Library of Congress Cataloging in Publication Data
Data available
ISBN 0-19-286166-2

10 9 8 7 6 5 4 3 2 1

Typeset by Pentacor PLC, High Wycombe, Bucks
Printed in Great Britain by
Clays Ltd.,
Bungay, Suffolk

Contents

Glossary of non-conventional therapies

A brief explanation is needed for the use of the terms 'complementary medicine' and 'non-conventional therapies' in this book. *Complementary medicine* is used in the title of this report, as it is the term which is most widely known by members of the public and other readers. However, the term *non-conventional therapies* is used hereafter in the text. This term is a more accurate description of the wide range of therapies covered in this book, which may be used both as alternatives and as complementary forms of treatment to orthodox medicine. A full discussion of the different terms in current usage is given in Chapter 1 for the information of the reader.

Given below are brief working definitions of the principal therapies covered in the BMA survey of non-conventional therapies. Readers wishing more detailed information on the practice or techniques of particular therapies should contact the organizations representing different therapies. The definitions used in this glossary have been formulated by the BMA, using the following three sources: information given in the BMA survey responses and accompanying literature from individual organizations; T. Smith (ed.), *British Medical Association Complete Family Health Encyclopedia* (Dorling Kindersley, London, 1990); and the *Readers Digest Family Guide to Alternative Medicine* (Readers Digest Association, London, 1991).

Acupuncture   Traditionally a branch of Chinese medicine, in which needles are inserted into the patient's body as therapy for various disorders or to induce anaesthesia.

Alexander technique Postural re-education by teaching people to stand and move more efficiently.

Aromatherapy Massage with external use of plant essential oils diluted in a base oil of vegetable origin.

Bach flower remedies Series of infusions made from wild plants, bushes, and trees, taken internally in diluted form.

Chiropractic Uses joint-adjusting procedures, manipulation, massage, and other techniques to treat musculo-skeletal complaints. Much emphasis placed on use of spinal X-rays for the diagnosis of mechanical problems.

Crystal therapy Healing by use of crystals, gems, and elixirs.

Healing To restore to health by non-physical means, often involving the 'laying on of hands'.

Herbalism Systems of treatment in which various parts of different plants are used in order to restore function and to treat symptoms.

Homoeopathy Treatment of patients by administering highly diluted forms of natural substances that in a healthy person would bring on symptoms similar to those which the medicine is prescribed to treat.

Hypnotherapy Inducing a state of hypnosis as a relaxation technique, to reduce pain and to bring about changes in mental state.

Iridology Method of diagnosis based on studying the markings on the irises of the eyes and observing changes in them.

Kinesiology Testing muscles to access information about the body. Using light touch or firm pressure on the reflex points of the body, together with diet, to restore balance.

Massage

Rubbing and kneading of areas of the body, normally using the hands.

Osteopathy

System of diagnosis and treatment whose main emphasis is on conditions affecting the musculo-skeletal system. Uses predominantly gentle manual and manipulative methods of treatment to restore and maintain proper biomechanical functions.

Radionics

Method of healing, using instrumentation to provide specific corrective energies to the patient through contact, medication, or broadcasting at a distance. Note: includes the practices of biomagnetics and signalysis therapy.

Reflexology

Compression and massage techniques using reflex points in hands and feet.

Shiatsu

Japanese form of massage, literally meaning 'finger pressure'. Uses pressure on hundreds of surface points of the body.

Introduction

> There are some patients whom we cannot help; there are none
> whom we cannot harm.
>
> Arthur L. Bloomfield (1888–1967)[1]

The British Medical Association (BMA) Board of Science and
Education was established to support the Association in its
founding aim 'to promote the medical and allied sciences and to
maintain the honour and interests of the medical profession'. Part
of the remit of the Board is to undertake research studies on key
public-health issues on behalf of the Association. Over the past
decade it has helped to formulate BMA policy on a wide range of
scientific and public-health issues, from smoking and road safety
to pesticide toxicity, infection control, and the environmental
effects of nuclear war. The objective of the Board is to provide
guidance to the profession and information to the public on
health-related issues which are of general concern, while influenc-
ing government and policy-makers. When endorsed by BMA
Council, its reports become Association policy. One such topic of
general professional and public interest is the different practices
loosely grouped together as non-conventional therapies.

Various indicators suggest an increase in the use of non-
conventional therapies over recent years. This is not a
phenomenon unique to the UK; a recent major survey from the US
estimated that one in three American adults had used some form of
non-conventional therapy in 1990,[2] which was a much higher
figure than previously reported. Different explanations have been
offered to account for this growth, from dissatisfaction with

conventional forms of treatment to more general theories of diversification of health care. This report does not attempt to assess the efficacy or validity of the different forms of non-conventional care available in the UK. The laws of this country ensure that, for the most part, adult citizens are entitled to make a choice as to the form of health care which they receive, and this system of regulation is unlikely to be changed in coming years.

It is not, therefore, the place of the medical profession to proscribe the legitimate activities of consumers in health care. However, doctors have a duty to the individual and to the community to safeguard the public health and, to this end, it is important that patients are protected against unskilled or un-scrupulous practitioners of health care. It was therefore considered helpful for the BMA to consider, as a *public-health* issue, the principles of good practice in non-conventional therapies which would safeguard the individual against possible harm to health and maximize the potential benefits of particular methods.

In 1986 the BMA produced a report, 'Alternative Therapy', which set out to investigate ways of assessing the value of different alternative therapies. Since 1985, the time at which evidence for the earlier report was collected, there have been a number of important developments in non-conventional therapies. Several issues which were not addressed in the earlier report feature prominently in the current debate: How widespread is the use of different therapies? Is the situation in the UK comparable to other countries in the EC? Do people consult therapists instead of or as well as seeing their doctor? How can patients be protected against incompetent practitioners?

A working-party was set up in 1990 by the BMA Board of Science and Education with the following terms of reference: 'to consider the practice and use of complementary medicine since 1985 throughout the UK and the European Communities and its implications after 1992.' This report follows from the working party's discussions.

Following a definition of non-conventional therapies at the beginning of the report, the second chapter reviews current and future legislative changes proposed for the Community and examines developments in the regulation of different therapies throughout Europe. Information was obtained from medical associations and ministries of health in different European countries. On examination of the evidence, the working-party concluded that the EC is unlikely to exert significant central control on the diverse practices of different countries. It seems probable that the most important influence on the regulation of non-conventional therapies will continue to be national law for the most part, rather than Brussels. Given this importance of UK law and regulation on the practice of non-conventional therapy in this country, the working party decided to focus its attention on recent developments in the UK.

Chapters 3 and 4 of this report provide background on the scope and nature of non-conventional therapies and the relationship between doctor and therapist in the UK. This includes a detailed examination of determining levels of competence in different therapies, highlighting areas of collaboration between the medical profession and different forms of non-conventional therapies, and an important discussion of the role of research and scientific enquiry in evaluating different forms of care. This is followed by debate on the possible options for regulation of non-conventional therapies, and the statutory regulation of osteopathy is considered as a case study.

The report concludes in Chapters 6 and 7 with the results of a national survey which was carried out by the British Medical Association to obtain detailed information from key bodies on the organization, ethical standards, training, qualification procedures, and research in various non-conventional therapies. On the basis of the helpful responses received from these bodies, the broad principles of good practice are discussed in each of these areas and set out in the last chapter. It is clear that there are many encouraging initiatives currently taking place in the field of non-conventional therapy, and it is hoped that good practice in each can be extrapolated for general use. The full summaries of the survey responses are given in the report for the information of the reader.

This report was prepared under the auspices of the Board of Science and Education of the British Medical Association, whose membership for 1992/3 was as follows:

Sir John Reid	*President, BMA*
Dr W. J. Appleyard	*Chairman of Representative Body, BMA*
Dr J. Lee-Potter	*Chairman, BMA Council*
Dr J. A. Riddell	*Treasurer, BMA*
Professor J. B. L. Howell	*Chairman, Board of Science and Education*
Professor J. P. Payne	*Deputy Chairman, Board of Science and Education*

Dr J. M. Cundy
Dr A. Elliott
Dr R. Farrow
Dr R. Gilbert
Dr L. P. Grime
Dr K. Hildyard
Dr A. Mitchell
Dr G. M. Mitchell
Col. M. J. G. Thomas, L\RAMC
Dr D. Ward

The Board of Science and Education was advised by a working party whose membership was as follows:

Professor J. P. Payne (Chair)	*Emeritus Professor of Anaesthesia, University of London*
Dr J. M. Cundy	*Consultant anaesthetist, Lewisham Hospital*
Dr M. Goodman	*General practitioner, Liverpool*
Professor T. W. Meade	*Director, Medical Research Council (MRC) Epidemiology and Medical Care Unit, London*
Dr G. M. Mitchell	*Consultant toxicologist, Cardiff*
Col. M. J. G. Thomas, L\RAMC	*Commanding officer, Army Blood Supply Depot*

Further assistance was given by Professor B. T. Williams and Dr D. T. Reilly.

1 Defining non-conventional therapies

1.1. What are non-conventional therapies?

In studying the practice and control of non-conventional therapies in the UK, the terminology is often unclear. What is understood by the phrase 'non-conventional therapies'? In a survey of general practitioners, the most common definitions of alternative medicine given were 'additional to western medicine' and 'not taught in medical schools'.[1] The World Health Organization (WHO) has defined alternative medicine as all forms of health-care provision which 'usually lie outside the official health sector'.[2] This global description by WHO embraces formalized traditional systems of medicine (Ayurvedic, traditional Chinese); traditional healers and medicine-men; biofeedback, chiropractic, naturopathy, osteopathy, homoeopathy, and 'even Christian science'. In the UK this definition would comprise more than sixty practices, including physical therapies such as osteopathy, psychological therapies such as hypnotherapy, and paranormal therapies such as healing. Indeed, Lord Skelmersdale, the Under-Secretary of Health, informed Parliament during a debate on complementary medicine in November 1987 that he had identified no fewer than 160 therapies, or variations of them.

The practices loosely grouped together under the umbrella of non-conventional therapies appear to have little in common, beyond the fact that they all 'treat' patients. A list of the principal therapies and a brief description of the methods used are given in the Glossary at the beginning of this report. The spectrum of non-conventional therapies includes diverse practices, ranging from the manual therapies such as osteopathy which are firmly based upon the study of orthodox medical sciences, to practices such as radionics, which involves the 'transmission of corrective energy patterns' to individuals. Such different therapies are therefore grouped together as non-conventional therapies not because of a commonality of principle or practice, but because they stand outside the parameters of that health care which is standardly available on the National Health Service.

1.2.   Alternative versus complementary therapies

It is worth briefly making the distinction between those therapies which are viewed as 'complementary' and those described as 'alternative'. 'Complementary' therapies are those which can work alongside and in conjunction with orthodox medical treatment. Within this category there is clearly a wide diversity of types of practice, which would include self-help therapies such as yoga; re-educational therapies such as the Alexander Technique; relatively non-invasive therapies such as healing and massage; and all interventive therapies such as acupuncture, osteopathy, and chiropractic. Practitioners such as osteopaths or chiropractors can, for example, treat the mechanical components of a musculo-skeletal problem whilst the patient is concurrently taking prescribed medications from their general practitioner, in the form of analgesics, non-steroidal anti-inflammatory drugs (NSAID), or muscle relaxants. In this role, the therapies are an additional and a complementary form of treatment. In the clinical practices of osteopathy and chiropractic, the basic training is largely grounded in the orthodox medical sciences and, as such, practitioners of these disciplines are able to have a close dialogue with their medical colleagues which is based upon a common language. Training modules for these practices increasingly place emphasis on working in conjunction and liaison with established health-care professionals.

By contrast, 'alternative' therapies could be seen as those which are given in place of orthodox medical treatment. While clearly any non-conventional therapy could in some circumstances be used as an alternative form of treatment—for example, if a practitioner of any discipline suggested that the patient should not receive concurrent orthodox medical treatment—there are some therapies which, by their very nature, aim to *replace* orthodox medicine. Examples of such therapies might include herbal medicines, which are often given in place of orthodox medication, as an alternative to allopathic drugs.

1.3. Medicine and non-conventional therapies

In answering the question: 'What are non-conventional therapies?' we therefore pose another question: 'What is conventional medicine?' The simple answer is, that treatment which is delivered by a registered medical practitioner. The 1858 Medical Act ensured that only practitioners registered with the newly established General Medical Council could practise conventional medicine or surgery. An attempt at the first reading of the Bill to prescribe the limits of medicine by including a clause outlawing the practice of 'unconventional' forms of therapy was rejected. It was thus permitted in law for doctors to practise whatever form of treatment they wished. Subsequent legislation, such as the 1946 National Health Act, similarly did not specify what *form* of treatment should be available on the National Health Service. Section 29(1) of the 1977 NHS Act lays down the duties and responsibilities of health authorities in providing medical services. There is currently no provision at this basic level for patients to seek treatment under the NHS directly from practitioners of non-conventional medicine.

1.4. Summary

There is no common principle linking the different non-conventional therapies. A review of the therapies listed in the glossary gives an indication of the diversity of philosophy and practice to be found in those techniques grouped together as non-conventional therapies. The working definition of non-conventional therapies used in this report is: *those forms of treatment which are not widely used by the orthodox health-care professions, and the skills of which are not taught as part of the undergraduate curriculum of orthodox medical and paramedical health-care courses.*

The terms non-conventional, complementary, unorthodox, alternative, natural, and fringe medicine are often used interchangeably. The phrase *non-conventional therapies* will be used in this report as a general and neutral term within which to explore the diverse nature of different practices.

2 Non-conventional therapies in Europe

2.1. Recent trends in Europe

There is a long history of official antagonism towards non-conventional medicine in many European countries, dating back to the last century when public authorities opposed its practice. Despite the implementation of many regulations, including the monopoly of medical practice for qualified doctors, the practice of non-conventional medicine persisted and grew in popularity, often simply because in rural areas it was the only form of health care available.

One of the main reasons for the current upsurge of 'official' interest in non-conventional medicine is the rapidly increasing number of patients who are seeking help from such practitioners. This has prompted the Council of Europe to state: 'It is not possible to consider this phenomenon as a medical side-issue. It must reflect a genuine public need which is in urgent need of definition and analysis.'[1]

There is no doubt that non-conventional and traditional forms of medicine are currently enjoying a renaissance throughout Europe. This increase in popularity had its birth in the 1960s with the advent of 'alternative' life-styles and was particularly popular with the younger section of the community, who have become increasingly concerned by environmental issues. The continuing popularity of non-conventional therapies has prompted many European countries to review their current policies. Evidence of use and increasing acceptance of non-conventional medicine is exemplified by several studies conducted in different European countries; for instance, a 1987 Netherlands study of general practitioners indicated that in 1981 3.8 per cent of the Dutch population had visited an 'alternative' medicine practitioner, and by 1987 this figure had risen to 5.2 per cent of the population.[2] The same study also suggested that 95 per cent of the respondents would discuss the option of alternative treatment with their patients and 90 per cent of the GPs referred patients for 'alternative' treatment, most commonly manipulation, homoeopathy, and acupuncture.

2.2.   The debate on harmonization

Regulation of the practice of non-conventional medicine within Europe is complex and somewhat confused. The advent of the single market and increasing desire for greater harmonization in the sale and delivery of products and services across national borders has led to suggestions of legislation at EC level governing the practice of non-conventional therapies in all member states of the European Community.

Over the last few years, considerable concern has been expressed by some groups of non-conventional therapists in the UK regarding the fate of complementary medical practice after the advent of the single market, which came into effect on 1 January 1993. The perceived antagonism in many EC countries towards the British style of 'unlicensed' practitioners of non-conventional medicine and the adoption of the General Systems Directive in December 1988 fuelled these anxieties. This Council Directive (89/48/EEC) provided mutual recognition of diplomas (or equivalent) awarded after training of at least three years' duration in a 'regulated profession'. As the practice of non-conventional therapy in the UK is not at present a professionally regulated activity or governed by a chartered body, the Directive simply does not apply to non-conventional practitioners in this country. A more recent directive (General System Directive CD/92/51) on the mutual recognition of professionals trained for less than three years has just been drafted which may have some bearing on non-conventional therapists.

As a result of the diversity and confusion that exists in relation to the practice of non-conventional therapies in Member States, the European Commission has chosen to distance itself from the situation. When pressed to express an opinion on the practice of non-conventional medicine within the Community, the Commission has consistently stated its view that central legislation is unlikely.[3] The British Government confirmed this stance in a statement by Baroness Hooper in the House of Lords in May 1990:

So far as the Government are aware there is no European Community legislation in prospect which would restrict the practice of natural therapy in this country or choice by the public in using such services . . . The Commission has repeatedly made it clear that at present it has no intention of introducing centralised legislation on the grounds that the fundamental divergence between member states' legislation in this area would make it difficult to envisage harmonisation at Community level.[4]

In 1988, in answer to a petition to the European Parliament[5] concerning the provisions to regulate professional activity in the field of natural medicine, the Commission stated that it was the responsibility of individual Member States to reconcile the practice of various types of medicine, so that traditional medicine and branches of 'Hippocratic natural medicine' (non-conventional therapies) may be used together for the benefit of the general public. This being the case, the Commission at present has no intention of proposing instruments to give natural medicine official recognition.[6]

The Commission has consistently stated its belief that the delivery of health care, including non-conventional therapies, is outside its remit. For instance, in an answer given by Mr Bangemann on behalf of the Commission in June 1990, it was stated that: 'The organisation of the provision of medical care falls entirely within the competence of the Member States. The Member States set the regulations for therapeutic procedures . . . The Commission does not propose taking action in the provision of natural medicine.'[7] The Commission clearly believes that it should be up to each Member State to establish its own legal framework regulating the practice of non-conventional medicines, and it seems almost certain that the practice of these professions will continue to be governed by national law in the foreseeable future.

The Commission does, however, take a stand regarding the use of the title 'Doctor of Medicine'. In response to a written question,[8] the Commission said that it does not consider it appropriate to award the title of 'Doctor of Medicine' to individuals without advanced medical training. This statement was in response to indications that Spain seemed to be prepared to award the title of 'doctor' to naturopaths and other professional practitioners of 'natural medicine'. The Commission pointed out that diplomas, certificates, and other evidence of formal qualifications in medicine required to pursue a medical profession are awarded only to persons who have acquired adequate knowledge as set out in Article 1 of the Directive EEC 75/363. However, the Commission has not adopted any criteria for awarding the title 'Doctor in Medicine' and it does not intend to put forward any such proposals. Concerning the possible consequences for other Member States if Spain were to recognize practitioners in natural medicine as Doctors of Medicine, Lord Cockfield, replying on behalf of the Commission, stated that it was the sole responsibility of Spain and the Commission would not compel other Member States to change their attitude to recognize the profession in question. The Commission itself took the view[9] that, in the absence of Directives regulating certain professions, each Member State will retain the right to fix minimum qualifications for the exercise of these professions on their own territory.

2.3. Dietary supplements, homoeopathy, and herbal medicines

European legislation in the future, however, is likely to have a pronounced effect on the availability of some natural medicines, such as homoeopathic and herbal remedies, and dietary supplements, including vitamins and minerals. The Commission's position is that they would like to see a common policy on all medicines within the single European Market. Already implementation of EC Directives[10] have removed from the market a large number of herbal medicines, many of which have been freely available in the UK for years.

It is expected that the EC Commission will issue draft regulations to cover all natural medicines, including vitamins, minerals, dietary supplements, and herbal products. The market for such products is substantial and rapidly growing, with estimates of sales within the EC totalling 1,000 million pounds, of which sales in the UK in 1990 were worth some 200 million pounds.[11] Harmonization at Community level, however, is likely to be difficult to achieve as in the UK, Germany, Denmark, and the Netherlands dietary supplements are sold in all types of retail outlets from pharmacists to supermarkets. In southern Europe, France, and Belgium, the situation is very different, as supplements are mainly classified as medicines and require product registration and are often subject to advertising restrictions. In line with other medicines, such products would become subject to rigorous testing and clinical trials. In some EC countries the sale of supplements is also limited to retail pharmacies, and in Spain and Italy supplements are widely prescribed by doctors, thus reducing the overall consumer market size.

A draft EC directive on dietary supplements is currently being prepared which may lead to the reclassification of vitamins, minerals, amino acids, fish-liver oils, and other nutrients as drugs rather than foods. These products, which are now marketed freely as foods with minimal restraints, would need to be registered and acquire a product licence before reaching retailers' shelves. There are also likely to be restrictions on the health benefits which can be claimed by products under current food-labelling regulations. A preliminary discussion paper released by the EC[12] stated that 'claims relating to the prevention, treatment or cure of disease' should be prohibited for 'diet integrators' such as herbal preparations or vitamins and health foods in line with other foodstuffs. The next round of consultation for the draft directive on dietary supplements should prompt useful discussion on the subject.

Homoeopathy presents particular difficulties for the EC Commission in its attempt to reconcile national rules on health products for the twelve member states of the Community. In some states homoeopathy is merely tolerated, whereas in others, such as France and Germany, it is recognized for reimbursement from health-insurance systems. This poses something of a quandary for the Commission as, in principle under the European Single Market, it should be possible to market products legally produced in any one member state in the other eleven.[13]

In early 1991 the Commission responded to a written question[14] asking if the Commission intended to put forward proposals on measures to ascertain the effectiveness of homoeopathic products. In its reply the Commission attempted to maintain a stance of neutrality, stating that it wished to avoid being drawn into a debate between the supporters and opponents of the efficacy of homoeopathy. The Commission emphasized that its proposals were designed first and foremost to protect consumers by ensuring the quality and safety of homoeopathic remedies, which would be distinguished from other medicines by their different labelling.

In December 1991 the Council of Ministers reached a common position on a proposed Directive to widen single-market legislation on medicinal products to include homoeopathic medicines. The manufacture, control, import, and export of homoeopathic drugs will now be subject to the provisions of the 1965 and 1975 Directives (65/65/EEC and 75/319/EEC). This will give EC consumers greater access to herbal and homoeopathic medicines that are manufactured and marketed in the Community, whilst providing guarantees on their quality and safety, although of course no attempt is made to assess the effectiveness of different products under this form of legislation.

A distinction is made under this legislation, as stated above, between homoeopathic products classified as totally harmless and all other homoeopathic products. A 'simplified' registration procedure is available for the former, which are defined as 'traditional homoeopathic medicinal products placed on the market without specific therapeutic indications in a pharmaceutical form and dosage which do not present a risk'.[15] A system of proof of therapeutic effect would be required for other homoeopathic medical products, in particular those marketed as being effective against specific complaints and those which consist of multiple or complex homoeopathic preparations. In September 1992 the European Parliament further modified this directive (Council Directive 92/73/EEC) so that only products of very high dilution (1 in 10^4) would qualify for the proposed simplified registration.

In the UK homoeopathic medicines have to date been subject to the same controls as traditional medicines under the 1968 Medicines Act. The EC Directive would affect this UK legislation by removing the requirement for 'harmless' homoeopathic products to demonstrate efficacy and by permitting a simplified form of registration for such products. Other developments which are being floated by the Commission are the possibility of a European homoeopathic pharmacopoeia and a move towards a Community-wide regimen for social-security refunding of the cost of homoeopathic services and medicinal products and the organization of officially recognized teaching of the subject.

2.4. Future developments in Europe

While there is unlikely to be legislative change on non-conventional therapies at an EC level, there has been much publicity of late concerning the present and likely future powers of the Commission to act in various spheres of interest. What impact does the debate over the Maastricht Treaty have for the control and practice of non-conventional therapies?

The Maastricht Treaty on Political Union was signed by representatives of European Community national governments on 7 February 1992. It amends previous treaties (the Treaty of Rome, 1957 and Single European Act, 1986), and expands the Community's powers. Policy on public health is contained in Article 129 of the Treaty. Although the Community has already undertaken health-related initiatives and adopted legislation relevant to the free movement of health professionals, it has never had a clear mandate to act in the area of public health.

The Commission does not have competence to intervene in the funding and administration of health-care systems in different EC countries. This position will not change with the implementation of the Treaty. However, the Article on public health makes the following general provision: 'The Community shall contribute towards ensuring a high level of human health protection by encouraging co-operation among member states and, if necessary, lending support to their action.' The impact of this Article for the practice of non-conventional therapies across Europe is probably limited. However, the Commission may be able to play a part in the monitoring and surveillance of non-conventional therapies in different European countries. It may be useful to collect information on a Europe-wide basis on changes in regulation and development of initiatives such as setting competences and standards for different therapies.

One development which has the potential to improve current levels of comparative information on non-conventional therapies in Europe is the proposed Council of Science and Technology (COST) project on 'unconventional medicine'. COST is based within the general secretariat of the Council of the European Communities in Brussels and aims to co-ordinate activities in the field of science and research across the Community by developing relevant multi-centre programmes.[16]

The project on non-conventional therapies was proposed by the Swiss government at the beginning of 1991 and the original draft has been revised by various bodies across Europe, including the Research Council for Complementary Medicine in the UK. It is anticipated that this proposal will be considered for ratification in 1993.

A five-year framework has been proposed for this project, which would consider the medical, social, cultural, psychological, legislative, and economic implications of non-conventional therapies across Europe. In the field of medical research, the project—which is still at the early stages of a draft proposal—aims to:

- facilitate competitive and fruitful research activities by the examination of literature sources, the setting-up of literature data bands, and the possibility of co-ordinating existing literature sources;

- document the levels of pre-clinical and clinical research for individual non-conventional procedures by means of critical reviews of available data;

- develop and evaluate procedures for demonstrating the efficacy of individual non-conventional procedures and establish an appropriate advisory service for researchers in the field;

- perform clinical studies into the effects, clinical efficacy, and safety of non-conventional therapies; and

- investigate the alleged working principles attributed to many non-conventional therapy forms.[17]

Many questions are still left unanswered at this stage of this research project, such as: Where are the designated research centres to carry out this work? How will they be accredited to carry out this project? What are the criteria with which to evaluate different therapies? Who will be co-ordinating these tasks across Europe? What are the working definitions of 'unconventional medicine'? However, this initiative should be nurtured as a positive way of promoting collaboration and exchanging information across national boundaries in Europe.

The diversity of practice and control in different countries has already been noted. Given the conclusion that legislation affecting the organization of health care, including the practice of non-conventional therapies, is unlikely to be forthcoming under EC law, the onus rests on individual countries and their systems of control.

2.5. Regulations governing non-conventional therapies in Europe

It is worth considering in some detail the present control of therapies in different countries. The BMA is grateful to its fellow medical associations in Europe and various ministries of health who provided much of the following information, in response to requests by the BMA Board of Science and Education for details of the control and practice of non-conventional therapies in different countries. There is a disparity in the length of the different accounts, as attention has been focused on new developments, particularly in the Netherlands, which have acted as catalysts for more general debate on the necessary restraints and regulations on non-conventional practitioners. Having studied the recent proposals for regulation in the Netherlands, representing the most 'radical' model of regulation, brief accounts are given of present practice in Germany and Scandinavia, followed by a description of current practice in the UK. The section concludes with a summary of the situation in those countries governed by the Napoleonic code of law.

2.5.1. Netherlands

As in many other European countries, the practice of all forms of medicine in the Netherlands is legally restricted at present to registered medical practitioners. However, the practice of non-conventional therapies by non-medically qualified practitioners is widespread, and pressure from the public is forcing the authorities to review the present regulations. Although technically illegal, non-conventional therapists have been tolerated for many years and the police take no action unless there is clear evidence of harm to patients. The increasing interest in non-conventional medicine has stimulated the Royal Dutch Medical Association (KNMG) to initiate discussions between non-conventional and orthodox medical practitioners, and the National Council for Health Care and the Council for Health are due to present their reports on 'alternative' and 'complementary' medicine in the near future.

At present, medical practice in the Netherlands is regulated by the Act on the Practice of Medicine (WUG). This Act stipulates that medically qualified doctors are the only persons qualified to practise medicine. However, a Bill is currently before the Dutch Parliament which, if passed, will change the law with regard to the provision of health care.

The Bill on Health Care Professions proposes that the present legal framework be replaced by a system of registration and protection of titles. This would alter radically the existing legislation governing the practice of health care and would allow patients to choose for themselves not only the type of medical treatment they receive but also from whom they obtain it. The Lower House approved the Bill in June 1992 and it is now being considered in the Upper House. It is expected that this process will be completed by the end of 1993. If approved by Parliament, the first sections of the Bill on Health Care Professions would probably come into force by 1994/5.

In principle, the system will deregulate medical care and the general ban on unauthorized medical practice will be lifted. However, statutory registers will be established by the government for those professions which it is deemed necessary to control in this way in the interests of safeguarding the public. Existing medical practitioners will be admitted to the registers once they have satisfied certain legal requirements. Most criteria for registration will relate to the training that an individual has received, and these standards of training required for registration will be enshrined in legislation. Once practitioners are registered under the new legislation, they will have the right to practise under a protected title, with the aim of assuring prospective patients that they are qualified to legally recognized standards in a particular field of health care.

The principle of the new Dutch legislation in relation to health care is that everyone in theory may offer medical care, but the government will supply guarantees that the practitioners providing care under a protected title are indeed genuinely qualified 'experts'. It will then be left to the patient to determine whether or not to engage the services of a practitioner recognized in this way.

Some forms of treatment, however, will fall outside the lifting of the general ban on the unauthorized practice of medicine. These treatments are principally those which could pose a potential risk to the health of the patient if they are not administered by fully qualified medical practitioners. The list is not exhaustive and can be extended, if necessary. Additions must satisfy two criteria: that there is a risk of considerable damage in the case of unqualified treatment, and secondly, that there is a real likelihood of unqualified persons practising in that area. The following appear as restricted actions under Article 36 of the Bill:

penetration of human tissue by incision;
treatment involving obstetrics;

catheterization and endoscopy;
the giving of injections and the puncturing of human skin;
the administration of anaesthetics;
the use of radioactive materials, radiation in treatment;
the use of electrical cardiography and defibrillators;
the administration of electro-convulsive therapy;
in-vitro fertilization and other interventive fertility treatments;
shattering of renal or ureteric stones.

Not all medical practitioners will be allowed to administer the above treatments, as the new legislation will explicitly require that a practitioner should have practical experience and be competent in administering the restricted treatments. For example, dentists will not usually be permitted to give general anaesthetics because they lack sufficient practical training in this area. If medical practitioners do administer any of the 'restricted treatments' without having gained the necessary expertise, they will run the risk of prosecution.

An important part of the new legislation attempts to set standards for the quality of health care provided by a 'recognized' practitioner. As the government will in effect be providing a guarantee that practitioners who work under a legally protected title have expertise in their particular field, those practitioners will be required to meet certain training requirements. The Dutch government believes that the introduction of these basic training requirements is a sound mechanism for ensuring that the quality of health care is maintained. In addition, the proposed legislation will provide for the possibility of registering certain categories of practitioners for limited periods only. Under such a system a practitioner would lose the right to work under a protected title if he or she has not practised for a number of years and has not subsequently undertaken a refresher course. The proposed legislation also contains provisions which could be used to compel medical practitioners to undertake postgraduate training courses and submit themselves to peer-review procedures.

Disciplinary regulations are also covered in the proposed legislation covering a number of professions, such as dentists, doctors, pharmacists, clinical psychologists, psychotherapists, midwives, and nurses, thus providing an important means of ensuring that the quality of professional care is maintained. This would supersede the Act on Medical Discipline of 1928 which makes doctors subject to an official disciplinary law. It is proposed that the Disciplinary Boards will include professional colleagues as well as 'jurists' so that the practitioner under investigation can be examined by his or her peers, who will decide whether or not the individual has provided the expected standard of health care. If the Disciplinary Board decides that the treatment provided falls short of the quality expected, the practitioner in question could face a number of penalties, including the ultimate sanction of deregistration, thus forfeiting the right to practise under a protected title.

While the new legislation will provide the government with effective ways of preserving the quality of health care, the professional medical organizations themselves will be charged with the important tasks of organizing supplementary training courses, the setting up of procedures for peer review, and the establishment of codes of professional conduct. The Dutch government believes that in this way the principles of self-regulation will be maintained.

Clearly, the proposed Dutch legislation will have profound implications for the practice of non-conventional medicine in the Netherlands. In order to register, professional groups such as acupuncturists, osteopaths, chiropractors, and homoeopaths will have to provide a clear professional profile of their scope of practice and skills.

The Dutch government has a very positive policy towards non-conventional medicine and, as a result of a report published by the State Committee on Alternative Medicine the Government has now instigated the following measures:

- the establishment of an information-and-documentation centre to serve the public in seeking reliable practitioners;

- the setting up of a fund of one million guilders (approximately £300,000) a year to stimulate studies into the efficacy of non-conventional therapies;

- the creation of appropriate curricula for non-conventional therapies to be offered by higher-education institutes and universities;
- the organization of projects to promote co-operation between registered medical practitioners and non-conventional therapists;
- the investigation of possibilities of creating a standardization of the quality and reliability of practitioners of non-conventional therapies;
- the provision of a permanent Advisory Board on non-conventional medicine incorporated within the National Council of Health Care;
- the formulation of acceptable methodology for research into non-conventional therapies.

At the request of the Dutch parliament a study is already being prepared on the cost-effectiveness of non-conventional medicine.

2.5.2. *Germany*

In Germany, *Heilpraktiker* (health practitioners), established under the Natural Therapy Act of 1939, are granted a state licence to treat any patient, utilizing a wide range of non-conventional therapies including homoeopathy, acupuncture, naturopathy, hydrotherapy, and manipulation. It is technically illegal for anyone who is not a registered medical practitioner or a *Heilpraktiker* to practise non-conventional medicine. Medical schools in Germany are now obliged to test students on their knowledge of non-conventional medicine.[18]

2.5.3. *Scandinavia*

The Scandinavian countries, like Germany, tend to take a relatively permissive view of the practice of non-conventional medicine. In Denmark non-conventional therapists can practise legally, although they are bound by the Medical Act which restricts their scope of practice. Non-medically qualified practitioners cannot, for example, treat infectious diseases, perform surgery, or prescribe drugs. There is also provision for sanctions to be taken against a practitioner whose treatment endangers or damages a patient.

Sweden, Norway, and Finland are not yet EC members, but are members of the European Free Trade Association (EFTA) group, which has signed an agreement with the EC to form a European Economic Area. This is likely to come into effect in July 1993 and, after that time, EFTA countries will be bound by most single-market legislation, including existing mutual recognition directives and legislation on medicinal products. Their positions with regard to non-conventional medicine can therefore be discussed here.

In Sweden, public health and medical personnel are those registered with the National Board of Health and Welfare. Such practitioners are defined under the Supervision of Health and Medical Personnel Act, and include doctors, dentists, nurses, midwives, and physiotherapists. Since 1989 Sweden also recognizes chiropractors who satisfy the standards laid down by the Council of Chiropractic Education. Anybody can offer services in health and medical care, although the management of certain conditions, such as cancer, diabetes, infections, epilepsy, and pregnancy, are prohibited by law. Non-medical practitioners are also not allowed to treat children under 8 years of age.

In Norway, under the Medical Act of 1936 anyone is permitted to undertake and give treatment to patients, subject only to limitations regarding the treatment of certain diseases, such as cancer, tuberculosis, and sexually transmitted diseases. However, surgical procedures may only be given by licensed physicians or dentists.

It is worth noting that both Denmark and Norway regard the insertion of acupuncture needles as surgical intervention which may only be performed by physicians or dentists. In Norway, however, a physician may delegate the responsibility for this task to other health-care personnel.

2.5.4. *Finland*

Finnish law does not recognize the practice of non-conventional medicine by anyone other than a registered medical practitioner. Non-conventional therapists are, however, popular with the public and tolerated by the authorities. The Ministry of Health and Social Affairs recognizes the increasing contribution of non-conventional medicine to Finland's health-care system and, since 1975, acupuncture has been accepted as part of orthodox medical practice and its study forms part of the medical curriculum.

2.5.5. *United Kingdom*

In the UK and Eire, non-medically qualified practitioners of non-conventional medicine are free to practise, whatever their level of training. However, such therapies have not been routinely available in state provision of health care. The Secretary of State for Health has a statutory duty to provide a comprehensive health service under the terms of the 1977 National Health Service Act. This includes a responsibility for safeguarding the health of the nation. By law, all 'medical' treatment given under the NHS must be given by a 'duly qualified medical practitioner'.

However, under the UK system of common law, anyone can practise as a non-conventional practitioner irrespective of whether or not he has undergone any form of training, providing that he does not infringe the Medical Act 1983 by implying that he is a registered medical practitioner, or use any of the other titles, such as 'dentist', which are protected by statute. Practitioners of non-conventional medicine are also prohibited from advertising treatments or remedies for a number of conditions, including cancer—under the terms of Section 4 of the Cancer Act 1939—tuberculosis, diabetes, glaucoma, and epilepsy. It is not, however, illegal for therapists actually to treat patients with these conditions. An exception is the case of sexually transmitted diseases, where there are restrictions on the *treatment* as well as the advertising of services under the Venereal Disease Act of 1917.

There are also restrictions on who may practise certain professions. Unqualified practitioners may not claim to be, or practise, as pharmacists, midwives, or dentists, or imply that they are a state-registered practitioner regulated by the Professions Supplementary to Medicine Act 1960. This Act covers the following professions: chiropodists, dietitians, medical-laboratory technicians, occupational therapists, physiotherapists, radiographers, and orthoptists (Section 1(2)).

The freedom for patients in the UK to seek treatment from anyone who claims to be able to provide it has a long tradition. An Act passed in 1511, the second year of Henry VIII's reign, was intended to reform the practice of medicine by eliminating 'unqualified' practitioners. However, as a result of the considerable pressure of public opinion, the king had to persuade Parliament to amend this Act in 1543 to allow anyone to practise. More recently, when the Medical Bill was first introduced to Parliament in 1858, it contained a provision to strike off any doctor who practised 'unconventional' forms of therapy. This clause was, however, rejected by both Houses of Parliament, and the final Act allowed doctors to utilize any form of treatment they chose, subject only to regulation by the General Medical Council.

What protection is offered to consumers under UK law from incompetent or unskilled therapists? Harm may arise from injury following treatment by a practitioner without adequate training; use of a therapy or application which is inappropriate or injurious to the condition of the patient; and failure of the practitioner to identify a problem requiring attention from a medically qualified practitioner. At present, individuals are protected by the tort-based common law of negligence. This provides for prosecution under the broad category of breach of 'duty of care' to the patient.

Homoeopaths, herbalists, and others administering medicinal products would also be liable under the 1985 European Directive on Product Liability (85/374/EEC) if the treatment proved 'defective'; the question of EC legislation covering homoeopathic and herbal products will be discussed later in this chapter. This EC Directive was implemented in the UK by Part I of the Consumer Protection Act 1987, which came into force on 1 March 1988. Under the terms of the Act, a product is considered defective if 'the safety of the product is not such as persons generally are entitled to expect'.

Other legislation which would cover individuals receiving treatment from non-conventional therapists include the 1968 Trades Description Act and general health-and-safety legislation such as the 1974 Health and Safety at Work, etc., Act and the more recent Control of Substances Hazardous to Health (COSHH) Regulations

1988. This latter piece of legislation imposes rigorous standards on those in contact with hazardous chemicals and body fluids which may be infectious; an acupuncturist reusing unsterilized needles for invasive procedures would therefore be liable under this legislation. The 1982 Supply of Goods and Services Act further requires individuals to deliver services with 'reasonable skills and care'. In terms of professional standards, there are at present no registering bodies in the UK equivalent to the General Medical Council for doctors or the United Kingdom Central Council for Nurses and Midwives (UKCC) for nurses, to which complaints may formally be lodged for users of non-conventional therapies.

2.5.6. *France, Belgium, and Italy*

The situation which exists in other European Countries which follow the Napoleonic code of law, where in essence any activity is forbidden unless specifically permitted by law, is very different from the UK model. In states such as France, Belgium, and Italy the practice of non-conventional medicine by anyone who is not a registered medical practitioner is outlawed, and occasionally therapists are prosecuted for the illegal practice of medicine. The irony is that in these countries the practice of non-conventional medicine is thriving and, for the most part, generally tolerated by the authorities.

While the practice of osteopathy in France is illegal, the teaching of osteopathy is within the law, and the number of training institutions is rapidly expanding. In France and Belgium, the practice of non-conventional medicine by registered medical practitioners is also widespread. France has approximately 10,000 doctors who regularly prescribe homoeopathic medicines, compared to the several hundred practising homoeopathic doctors in the UK.

2.6. Summary

There is at present a great diversity in the practice and control of non-conventional therapies across Europe. There is a wide spectrum from, on the one hand, the liberal approach of the

Netherlands in particular and also the Scandinavian countries, to the more restrictive approach in the regulation of therapies in France, Belgium, and Italy. The situation is confused by the fact that in those latter countries where the practice of non-conventional therapy is restricted by law, the use of such therapies is in fact widespread. The UK sits midway on this spectrum; while unlicensed therapists are free to practise, such treatment is not standardly available on the National Health Service.

Given the heterogeneity of practice across Europe, it is unlikely that central control will be exerted from Brussels to regulate non-conventional therapies. However, European legislation will have a marked influence on the availability of homoeopathic and herbal medicines, although even in this defined area the diversity of use and definition of medicines in different countries may challenge the uniformity of such an approach. It is clear that the most important influence on the regulation of non-conventional therapies will continue to be national law, although directives from Brussels will have a marked effect on various areas, such as medicinal products. A mechanism for the exchange of information on non-conventional therapies in different European countries would be helpful in pulling together these diverse strands.

3 *Setting the scene in the UK*

3.1. Patterns of consultation and practice

It is very difficult at present to ascertain the numbers of non-conventional therapists in the UK. Existing figures are estimates based on surveys—including samples culled from the 'yellow pages' of telephone directories as well as from representative bodies—or data on selective therapies only. In 1981 Fulder estimated that there were around 30,000 practitioners, of whom 11,164 were in professional organizations.[1] If healers and practitioners of the creative therapies are excluded from Fulder's tally, then the estimate of therapists belonging to professional organizations was at that time around 4,000 individuals.

However, these data are more than ten years old, and evidence points to an exponential growth in the number of therapists in the last decade. Indeed, the British Holistic Medical Association estimates that the number of therapists is increasing at a rate of 11 per cent a year.[2]

A study by Fulder and Munro in 1985 projected that nationally there were twelve practitioners per 100,000 population.[3] Other recent attempts to document the number of practitioners include a survey by K. J. Thomas and colleagues published in 1991.[4] On the basis of their sample, the authors estimated that there were about 1,900 practitioners of acupuncture, chiropractic, homoeopathy, naturopathy, and osteopathy in Great Britain in 1987. This figure is likely to be a conservative estimate; results from the 1991 BMA survey, discussed in Chapter 6, indicate that membership of two major representative bodies for acupuncture and osteopathy alone exceeds 3,000.

In terms of uptake of non-conventional therapies, figures from the Consumers Association suggest an increase since 1985, when one in seven of their 28,000 members surveyed had visited some form of non-conventional therapist in the preceding twelve months. In 1991 that figure had increased to one in four, although it should be noted that these rates cannot be extrapolated to the general population given the unrepresentative nature of the Consumers Association sample. In this survey the therapies most commonly used, in order of popularity, were osteopathy, chiropractic, homoeopathy, and acupuncture, followed by aromatherapy, reflexology, and herbal medicine.[5] Indeed, in this survey osteopathy accounted for 40 per cent of all consultations.

Different projections are given for the total number of consultations nationally in the various branches of non-conventional therapy. Discrepancies in the figures cited below arise because of differences in the method of estimating the volume of consultations; some investigations have simply asked practitioners how many consultations they held, whereas others have examined records of the consultations. Fulder and Munro estimated that there were nationally 11.7 million – 15.4 million consultations a year; they also calculated that 1.5 million people (2.5 per cent) of the population received some form of non-conventional therapy during the course of a year. As a comparison, it is estimated that about 72 per cent of the population consult their general practitioner during the course of a year.[6]

The British Holistic Medical Association estimated that there were approximately 4 million consultations a year,[7] although their figures related only to therapists affiliated to the General Council and Register of Osteopaths (GCRO) or the Council for Complementary and Alternative Medicine (CCAM). On the basis of Thomas and colleagues' study of patients of practitioners of five non-conventional therapies with a regulatory body, the authors estimated that 70,600 patients are seen nationally for the therapies of acupuncture, chiropractic, homoeopathy, naturopathy, and osteopathy.[8] One study of homoeopathic doctors suggested a figure of 750,000 consultations a year of doctors by patients in the

UK yielding homoeopathic prescriptions.[9] Another study of general practitioners in Oxfordshire suggested that 5 per cent of all patients presenting to GPs had been treated by some form of non-conventional therapy.

The figures given are fairly imprecise but point to a considerable and growing number of people consulting non-conventional therapists. What sort of people are most likely to make use of non-conventional therapies? Latest figures from the General Household Survey show that consultation rates with general practitioners are highest among the elderly and children under 5 years of age.[10] By contrast, non-conventional therapists tend to treat individuals in their middle years.[11] Similarly, the greatest volume of work-load for general practitioners is derived from those in unskilled manual classes, who also have the highest rates of reported chronic sickness;[12] however, individuals attending non-conventional therapists appear to be drawn predominantly from social classes I and II, particularly for the more 'rarefied' therapies such as homoeopathy.[13] In the study by Thomas and colleagues two-thirds of the patients were women;[14] similar figures are given in the Fulder and Munro survey.[15] Regional trends show a preponderance of consultations in London and the south-east.[16] It can therefore be seen that the patterns of consultation appear to be different for 'conventional' and non-conventional practitioners.

3.2. Use of non-conventional therapies

Do people consult non-conventional therapists instead of seeing their general practitioner? In the survey by Thomas and colleagues of 2,473 patients seeking treatment with the therapies already noted, 64 per cent had received previous care from a general practitioner or hospital service.[17] The vast majority of this sample (78 per cent) were attending with musculo-skeletal problems—this could be attributed in part to the fact that two out of the five therapies in the survey were manipulative techniques. Interestingly, 22 per cent of the patients surveyed had seen their GP in the two weeks before consultation. This is higher than the average national figure of GP consultations; data from the nationally representative sample for the latest General Household Survey indicated that 11 per cent of males and 16 per cent of females had consulted GPs in the two weeks before the interview.[18] In addition, 24 per cent of the patients in the study by Thomas and colleagues were receiving concurrent orthodox treatment, in particular patients reporting atopic conditions (asthma, hay-fever), head-aches, and arthritis. The authors concluded that: 'Non-orthodox treatment was sought for a limited range of problems and used most frequently as a supplement to orthodox medicine.'[19]

The earlier study by Fulder and Munro similarly suggested 'dual and simultaneous models of health care' in which therapies were used as a complement to orthodox medicine.[20] In their study, 33.4 per cent of individuals seeking consultations from non-conven-tional therapists were simultaneously receiving help from medical practitioners. A smaller two-stage study by Murray and Shepherd of the prevalence and use of non-conventional therapies in a south London practice confirmed that 'the additional rather than exclusive use of alternative measures was the norm'.[21] The findings of this study suggested that patients consulted both the GP and the non-conventional practitioner for the same illness episode, so that increasing use of non-conventional therapies would not neces-sarily result in a reduction in the demand for GP services.

Interesting questions are raised regarding the nature of consulta-tions and the relation between doctors and 'lay' practitioners. Fulder and Munro argue that conventional and non-conventional therapists have discrete spheres of influence. Individuals consult-ing the latter tend to suffer from chronic, mild, musculoskeletal and stress-related conditions rather than acute, malignant, or infective diseases. This would suggest that the areas of operation are distinct and well delineated between orthodox medicine and non-conventional therapy, although these boundaries can at times be blurred.

Before discussing in detail the relationship between doctor and therapist, it is worth considering briefly the views and outlook of medical practitioners on non-conventional therapies.

3.3.   Medical interest in non-conventional therapies

Interest in non-conventional therapies over recent years has been evident among both the general public and the medical profession. A number of recent studies testify to the growing interest of doctors in non-conventional therapies, both in response to patients requesting information on various therapies and as a result of professional interest in different therapies. One of the most comprehensive enquiries into doctors' attitudes to and relations with non-conventional therapists was published in 1986 in the *British Medical Journal*. Wharton and Lewith[22] conducted a study using a random sample of 200 general practitioners in Avon, and received a 75 per cent response-rate of 145 GPs. The authors included in their definition of complementary medicine acupuncture, homoeopathy, herbalism, spinal manipulation, faith healing, and hypnosis. In the survey, 38 per cent of respondents claimed to have received training in some form of complementary medicine, principally in the form of weekend courses; a further 15 per cent wished to arrange training.

GPs perceived their own levels of knowledge as low; spinal manipulation was best understood (45 per cent) and herbalism the least understood (only 5 per cent claiming at least moderate knowledge) of these therapies. Reported poor levels of knowledge were confirmed by open questions where responses revealed gaps in understanding; the authors stated that many respondents, for example, appeared to think that acupuncture could be used to treat any condition. However, there were high levels of acceptance of these therapies, especially for spinal manipulation, which was acknowledged as useful or very useful by 89 per cent of respondents, followed by hypnosis (79 per cent), acupuncture (67 per cent), homoeopathy (47 per cent), healing (46 per cent), and herbalism (23 per cent).

In surveying the attitude of these GPs, 70 per cent thought that the 'most acceptable' techniques—acupuncture, spinal manipulation, homoeopathy, and hypnosis—should be available on the NHS. Only 3 per cent thought that the practice of these therapies by non-medically qualified practitioners should be banned, but 93 per cent agreed that non-medical practitioners required regulation. It was interesting to note that younger GPs were 9 per cent more likely than their older colleagues to delegate care of patients to non-conventional therapists.

The greater degree of support which appears to be present among younger physicians was confirmed by an earlier survey of GP trainees by Reilly.[23] Of the eighty-six trainees surveyed, eighteen used at least one alternative method while as many as seventy wished to train in one or more technique. Thirty-one trainees had delegated care to lay practitioners, most commonly to those practising hypnosis, manipulative techniques, homoeopathy, and acupuncture. Twenty-two had been treated by a non-conventional therapist themselves. Like the earlier study, the support given to different therapies was mirrored by the extent of reported knowledge in different areas; herbalism was rated useful by only 13 per cent of respondents compared to acupuncture (76 per cent) and hypnosis (74 per cent). A more recent study in 1987 by Reilly of 242 GP trainees suggested a maintained and indeed increasing level of interest in non-conventional therapies, with 92 per cent claiming some form of foundation course on the basis and use of different therapies.[24]

Much interest in studying the attitudes and practices of doctors towards non-conventional therapists has centred on general practice. The general practitioner occupies a special place in medicine, as the 'gatekeeper' for access to medical services. In discussing attitudes of medical practitioners to non-conventional therapists, it is interesting to note the results of a very large survey of GPs which was undertaken by the General Medical Services Committee in February 1992[25] as a comprehensive information-gathering exercise on all aspects of working and professional practice. Questionnaires were received from 25,458 general practitioners, representing 70 per cent of all registered GPs in the UK. In the survey, respondents were also asked which services —including hypnotherapy, homoeopathy, acupuncture, chiropractic, and osteopathy—they thought should be provided at GP surgeries in the future, assuming that adequate resources were made available. A full list of the responses is given in Table 3.1.

TABLE 3.1 Views of general practitioners as to which services should be provided at GP surgeries (%)

Service	Provided at GP surgeries?		
	yes	no	no strong view
Crisis counselling (eg. divorce, bereavement) (N=24,774)	68.8	15.2	16.1
Addiction counselling (eg. alcohol, drugs) (N=24,539)	54.9	26.5	18.6
Hypnotherapy (N=24,093)	22.9	41.9	35.2
Homoeopathy (N=24,052)	17.8	50.1	32.1
Acupuncture (N=23,986)	29.2	36.3	34.5
Dietetics (N=24,462)	79.7	8.9	11.4
Physiotherapy (N=24,575)	88.5	5.9	5.7
Chiropody (N=24,317)	80.0	9.6	10.4
Chiropractic (N=28,836)	21.4	42.4	36.2
Osteopathy (N=23,865)	29.1	37.5	33.4
Laboratory analysis/pathology (N=24,106)	41.2	38.0	20.8
Full pharmacy service (i.e. including over-the-counter drugs) (N=24,226)	32.6	45.8	21.6
Optometry (N=24,011)	35.1	35.0	29.9
Hospital consultant sessions (N=24,388)	58.9	20.4	20.7
X-ray services (N=24,143)	28.2	51.9	19.9
Endoscopy (N=24,220)	29.6	45.2	25.2

Source: Survey by General Medical Services Committee (1992).

It can be seen that although 29 per cent of respondents believed that acupuncture and osteopathy should be provided at GPs' surgeries, nearly 37 per cent believed that it was inappropriate to provide these services. The other non-conventional therapies listed received less support, with homoeopathy receiving the greatest opposition. It is interesting to note that a large proportion were undecided, with approximately a third of respondents having no strong view for each of the five non-conventional therapies. This latter fact may reflect the lack of reliable information on various aspects of non-conventional medicine, which may make it difficult for GPs and others to hold a firm view on the desirability of offering these services.

When analysing responses by age and gender a slightly different picture emerges. Younger GPs were more likely to support the inclusion of such therapies in general practice, with about a third of GPs under 45 years of age supporting the provision of acupuncture and osteopathy at GP surgeries, as opposed to less than a fifth of respondents over the age of 65 years. Women doctors were more likely to advocate inclusion of non-conventional therapists into general practice. There was also marginally greater support from fund-holders, but no difference in the views held by those working in urban and rural practices.

A more positive picture of support for non-conventional therapies by GPs emerges from a much smaller survey of 282 GPs by the journal *Doctor* in July 1992.[26] In this survey, 90 per cent of respondents believed that acupuncture was effective, and similar high levels of support were accorded to osteopathy (84 per cent), hypnotherapy (81 per cent), homoeopathy (80 per cent), and chiropractic (78 per cent). Only herbalism received more guarded support, with just over half believing it to be effective. The question of bias cannot be eliminated in this survey, however, as details of response-rate and other features of the methodology were not reported.

A study by Anderson and Anderson[26] of 222 GPs in Oxfordshire showed high levels of interest and use of non-conventional therapies. Of the doctors surveyed, 41 per cent believed that alternative systems of medicine were valid; 31 per cent of those surveyed claimed a working knowledge of at least one therapy and 59 per cent of respondents had delegated care of patients to lay practitioners; 12 per cent had received training and a further 41 per cent had attended lectures or classes; 42 per cent of respondents wanted more training in non-conventional therapies. It is interesting to note that in this study 95 per cent of the respondents stated that patients had discussed non-conventional therapies with them during the past year.

The responsibilities of medical practitioners and their relationship with non-conventional therapists pose a number of interesting questions. Some of the key points will be addressed in Chapter 4, in which a general overview is given of the present position of those therapies outside the parameters—or on the margins—of the health service. The complex issues which are raised may not result in clear answers, but in identifying some of the problems it is hoped that further discussion of these important questions will be catalysed.

3.4.   Summary

There are a wide range of non-conventional therapies which are currently practised in the UK. Reliable data are not available on the extent and scope of the different therapies, although what information exists suggests a growing number of therapists and an increase in the number of people seeking help from different non-conventional therapies. Currently available information suggests that the therapies most commonly used are acupuncture, the manipulative therapies—osteopathy and chiropractic—herbal medicine, and homoeopathy.

From existing—incomplete—data, a picture can be built up of patterns of consultation. The greatest work-load for general medical practitioners is derived from the very old and the very young and from those in the unskilled manual classes. This contrasts with patients presenting to non-conventional therapists, who are more likely to be middle-aged, female, and from social classes I and II. There also appear to be marked regional trends in the prevalence of non-conventional practice, as many therapists are concentrated in London and the south-east.

There is growing interest among medical practitioners in various non-conventional therapies; this is particularly marked in younger doctors and in women doctors. One survey suggested that interest was sufficient to stimulate training in some form of therapy amongst a third of GPs. Whether or not doctors wish to practise different techniques themselves, it is clear that there is a definite need among doctors for better *information* in the use and practice of non-conventional therapies, which is not presently being met.

4 Therapies and the medical profession

4.1. Doctors and therapists

Individuals may consult a non-conventional therapist of their own volition, or following the advice of their doctor. The vast majority of consultations are 'self-referrals' by patients, that is, individuals going directly to a therapist for treatment. This point should be borne in mind during the course of this chapter, as the proportion of patients seeing a therapist as a result of the recommendation of their doctor is still relatively small. However, anecdotal evidence from the General Medical Council and others suggest that doctors are increasingly asking for advice about different therapies, as a growing number of clinicians wish to make use of such services for their patients.

To date there is a paucity of reliable data on the extent to which doctors delegate care to non-conventional therapists. In the study by Wharton and Lewith, a high proportion of the doctors surveyed (71.7 per cent) had delegated care of patients to therapists; younger GPs were 9 per cent more likely than their older counterparts to delegate care to lay practitioners.[1] Anderson and Anderson's study of GPs suggested similarly that more than half of those surveyed had 'referred'(*sic*) patients to non-conventional therapists.[2] In the study of GP trainees, 36.1 per cent had delegated care of patients to therapists, most commonly for hypnosis, manipulation, homoeopathy, and acupuncture.[3] These studies may not be representative of all general practitioners but suggest that, to a greater or lesser degree, general practitioners are delegating care to non-conventional therapists.

Under the provisions of the 1858 Medical Act, a doctor could be removed from the register for sending a patient to a practitioner who was not medically qualified. This remained the official position until fairly recently. Guidance from the General Medical Council in 1969 specified that 'any doctor who knowingly enables or assists a person, not duly qualified and registered as a medical practitioner, to practise Medicine or to treat patients in respect of matters requiring medical or surgical discretion or skill, becomes liable to disciplinary proceedings'.[4] However, the part played by nurses, midwives, physiotherapists, radiographers, and other non-medically qualified health-care workers is now well recognized by the medical profession. The General Medical Council in Paragraphs 42 and 43 of the latest version of its guidance for doctors, *Professional Conduct and Discipline: Fitness to Practise* (April 1992), sets out the conditions of the delegation of medical duties to nurses and others:

42.   The Council recognises and welcomes the growing contribution made to health care by nurses and other persons who have been trained to perform specialised functions, and it has no desire either to restrain the delegation to such persons of treatment or procedures falling within the proper scope of their skills or to hamper the training of medical and other health students. But a doctor who delegates treatment or other procedures must be satisfied that the person to whom they are delegated is competent to carry them out. It is also important that the doctor should retain ultimate responsibility for the management of his patients because only the doctor has received the necessary training to undertake this responsibility.

43.   For these reasons a doctor who improperly delegates to a person who is not a registered medical practitioner functions requiring the knowledge and skill of a medical practitioner is liable to disciplinary proceedings . . .

The distinction between delegation and referral of care has not always been clear. In considering the relationship between non-conventional therapists and medical practitioners, the working party has made distinctions between the modes of referral and delegation. The use of these terms for the purpose of this report is outlined below.

Referral can be used to describe a situation where one medical practitioner refers a patient to another doctor for an additional opinion or specialized treatment. A doctor can also refer a patient to a non-medically qualified practitioner, such as a dentist, or indeed a non-conventional therapist of one of the discrete clinical disciplines (see Chapter 5) for medical treatment or care which falls outside the scope of the medical care normally provided by the doctor him- or herself. The doctor refers a patient to another individual to use his or her professional judgement to assess the patient and decide if (and what) treatment is necessary and, where appropriate, to provide that treatment. In the referral model, the general practitioner refers care of the patient to a specialist for a particular episode of treatment, but will retain clinical responsibility for the overall care of the patient. In the words of the General Medical Council: 'The medical profession in this country has always considered that it is in the best interests of patients for one doctor to be fully informed about and responsible for the comprehensive management of a patient's medical care' (Paragraph 92).

By contrast, in delegating care, the general practitioner asks another professional to perform a specific function or provide medical treatment or care which might otherwise be carried out by the doctor and for which the doctor remains clinically accountable. For instance, a doctor may delegate the giving of an injection or the taking of a blood sample to a nurse in this way. In this case, a specific task which is routinely performed by the doctor is delegated to another health professional. The fact that the doctor takes overall responsibility of course does not remove the onus from the nurse or other practitioner to judge whether they are competent to carry out the task. These different kinds of responsibility and other general issues of inter-professional relations are discussed further in the BMA report on medical ethics.[5]

It is clearly the responsibility of the doctor who delegates care in this way to ensure that the individual practitioner to whom care is delegated is competent in the therapy practised. This is relatively straightforward in the case of a therapy which has been subject to statutory regulation for some time, such as nursing (dates of state registration for the following professions are: medicine, 1858; midwifery, 1902; nursing, 1919; dentistry, 1921). Problems do arise when there is no central register for a particular therapy and no single accrediting body for training and qualification. Indeed, this was the problem facing the medical profession prior to the passage of the 1858 Act. It should be noted that, prior to the publication and approval of the Act by Parliament, no fewer than *twenty* medical Acts had been introduced abortively into Parliament; its passage was not an easy one.

John Simon, who introduced the 1858 Bill as Medical Officer of the General Board of Health from 1855 to 1858, stated the reasons why such legislation was necessary, citing first the fragmentary nature of the medical profession—or professions, given the differing claims and outlooks of the physicians, surgeons, and apothecaries. One of his chief concerns was that 'titles purporting to certify the medical attainments of their bearers' could be obtained from twenty-one different sources within the UK, including the Archbishop of Canterbury. He stated:

These titles are given entirely without concert among the several institutions which award them, and without responsibility to any common authority. They represent twenty one different standards, each fixed and varied at the discretion of the authority which applies it, of what is the minimum knowledge wherewith a candidate may properly be allowed to practise part or all of his profession.[6]

This description tallies to a certain extent with the picture of non-conventional therapies today. Later in the report consideration will be given to the need for common standards of training and competency in order to establish the individual's 'fitness to practise'. It is clear, however, that given the current situation in this country in which there is only partial registration, the validation of bona-fide therapists is not easy for the patient/client or for a doctor who may delegate care. (Even after the establishment of a system of statutory registration which involves some form of 'grandfather' clause—allowing long-standing practitioners without formal qualifications but with considerable experience to practise—careful judgement will need to be exercised in choosing an appropriately qualified therapist. Only after a number of years have elapsed can it be certain that the majority of practitioners will have been trained to the same high standards of competence.) Before considering in detail the process by which doctors delegate care to non-conventional therapists, it is worth reviewing briefly the special case of doctors who themselves practise some form of therapy.

4.2. Doctors as therapists

It is difficult to ascertain the number of medically qualified individuals practising some form of non-conventional therapy. The category of medically qualified practitioner may embrace a broad range of activities, from a doctor employing homoeopathic skills on a fairly full-time basis to the doctor practising hypnotherapy on patients very occasionally. Fulder estimates that there are around 2,000 doctors practising non-conventional therapies.[7] Sixteen per cent of the sample of general practitioners surveyed by Anderson and Anderson claim to practise a form of 'alternative medicine', although this figure cannot necessarily be extrapolated to the population of doctors at large. It was of some concern that nine of the doctors in the survey by Anderson and Anderson appeared to have received no formal training in the therapies mentioned, which included the interventive therapies of manipulation and acupuncture as well as the more 'passive' modes of healing, hypnosis, and transcendental meditation.

A number of organizations already exist for doctors actively practising and qualified in different non-conventional disciplines. The Faculty of Homoeopathy is a long-established postgraduate and professional body, set up in 1844 for doctors practising homoeopathic medicine which has about 250 practising members. Similarly, the British Osteopathic Association has a membership of approximately seventy-five doctors and the British Medical Acupuncture Society has approximately 300 members who are all doctors practising acupuncture. There is also a British Society of Medical and Dental Hypnosis which has about 600 practising members who are all medically qualified.

Nurse practitioners are involved in increasing numbers in training in different non-conventional therapies or adjunctive techniques. Courses on massage, nutrition, aromatherapy, reflexology, and counselling now figure as part of different nursing curricula. The Royal College of Nursing has set up a Special Interest Group in Complementary Therapy for nurses active in research in some branch of non-conventional therapy.[8]

It should be noted that very clear advice is given by the General Medical Council regarding responsibility of the doctor for standards of medical care. While medical practitioners are free to practise whatever form of medicine is appropriate to the patient, there are stringent requirements to achieve the basic qualifying standards of medical competency and knowledge in the application of whatever branch of medicine or technique they practise. A medically qualified practitioner remains accountable to the General Medical Council whatever treatment he or she is undertaking. Paragraph 38 of the standard GMC guidance sets out the following as a condition of serious professional misconduct: 'persisting in unsupervised practice of a branch of medicine in which he does not have the appropriate knowledge and skill and has not acquired the experience which is necessary'. It is clearly unsatisfactory for medical practitioners who have received little formal training to undertake therapies for which they are not competent. Where there are clear and recognized standards of competence laid down for a therapy, such as osteopathy, the therapist, whether medically qualified or not, should satisfy those criteria.

The position in terms of referring patients from doctor to doctor-therapist is similarly clear. As set out in the 1988 BMA handbook of ethics for doctors,[9] the position of a medically qualified hypnotist or acupuncturist in general practice is analogous to that of a specialist in relation to patients not on their list. As a specialist, the practitioner must observe the GMC guidance of not proceeding with treatment—except in emergencies—until the patient's own GP has been contacted. In the case of a self-referral in which patients approach the medically qualified therapist themselves, the GP could only be contacted with the consent of the patient. The patient's consent, however, is not needed in the case of a referral of a patient from a doctor to a medically qualified therapist.

Homoeopathy occupies a special place in relation to the NHS and the wider medical profession. In 1950, following an 'absolute guarantee' by the Minister of Health in 1949 that homoeopathy would be allowed to continue within the National Health Service for as long as patients demanded it, the Faculty of Homoeopathy Act was passed. This Act provided for the incorporation of the Faculty, as a postgraduate training establishment for doctors, with the objective of 'advancing and extending the principles and practice of homoeopathy'.[10] There are currently six NHS homoeopathic hospitals in the UK, usually practising a mixture of homoeopathic and orthodox techniques. A survey by Swayne of members of the Faculty of Homoeopathy indicated that of a total of 7,218 consultations, 88 per cent were part of the NHS.[11] It is perhaps paradoxical to note that homoeopathy which, in many ways, acts as an alternative mode of treatment to allopathic medicine, is the only therapy to fall formally under the aegis of the NHS.

Medically qualified therapists comprise a small but significant proportion of all non-conventional therapists. Other medically qualified practitioners make use of various therapies without practising themselves; this is done by utilizing the services of a non-conventional therapist. It is worth scrutinizing a little more closely the process by which patient care is transferred from a doctor to a non-medically qualified therapist.

4.3. Use of therapies in the NHS

In a parliamentary statement of December 1991, the Parliamentary Secretary of State for Health attempted to clarify the position of alternative and complementary therapies within the NHS. The minister stated that 'alternative therapies' could be delivered either by doctors themselves, or treatment could be delegated to therapists who remain clinically accountable to the registered medical practitioner responsible for the patient's care.

General practitioners are self-employed individuals who enter into contracts with Family Health Services Authorities (FHSAs) in England and Wales and Health Boards in Scotland and Northern Ireland to provide general medical services. They have always been able to employ whatever staff they considered appropriate to assist them in the provision of these services, subject to certain limitations. However, with the introduction of the new contract from 1 April 1990, restrictions on the numbers and types of staff for whom GPs could claim direct reimbursement from their FHSAs/Health Boards have been removed. Under the new Practice Staff Scheme there is no longer a definition of 'qualifying staff', and thus a GP may claim payments for a wider range of staff, including, for example, physiotherapists, chiropodists, dietitians— and osteopaths and other non-conventional therapists.[12] These changes were accompanied by amendments in April 1992 to the 'Terms of Service for Doctors in General Practice' which are enshrined in legislation. Under Paragraph 28 of these regulations, before employing anyone to assist in the provision of general medical services GPs are required to take reasonable care to satisfy themselves that such persons are both suitably qualified and competent to discharge the duties for which they are employed.[13] Essentially, therefore, it is a matter for the judgement of the GP to ascertain the appropriateness of delegation of patient care to a non-conventional therapist.

Within the NHS, GPs may 'employ' a complementary therapist to offer treatment in the GP's surgery or in the therapist's own practice setting. In order to do this, the GP would make a bid for individual posts or sessions to his or her FHSA/Health Board. The authority has discretion to pay all, part, or none of these costs. It has been pointed out that the need for extra nursing and clerical staff to implement the new contract, together with the cash limits imposed on FHSAs and Health Boards, may in practice deter GPs from employing 'additional' staff such as acupuncturists, osteopaths, or counsellors.[14] Greater discretion is of course afforded to fund-holding GPs who can transfer additional resources from another part of the fund for the employment of ancillary professional staff, without requiring the prior approval of the FHSA or Health Board.

Flexibility is given, therefore, to both fundholders and nonfundholders, not only in the amount of NHS reimbursement for non-conventional therapies but also in terms of the 'employment' of non-conventional therapists. For many GPs, however, who wish to delegate care to therapists, it may not be practicable to employ such staff within their own practices. For instance, it may not be possible, given restriction of finances and space, for the GP to accommodate chiropractors or osteopaths with specialist equipment such as hydraulic manipulative tables. Given the changes in general practice outlined above, it seems likely that primary health-care teams will be expanding in coming years, with the development of multi-disciplinary teams of GPs and nurses, as well as dietitians, physiotherapists, counsellors, and others. There is likely, therefore, to be increasing pressure on practice facilities and resources. For these reasons, it may be preferable for the GP to employ therapists working from other premises.

Another factor is the need for support and peer review for practitioners of these therapies themselves; it has been noted that there has been an exponential increase over the last ten years in the demand for various therapies and a corresponding growth in the number of practitioners. In some therapies, over half of those practising have been graduated for less than ten years. For example, membership of the General Council and Register of Osteopaths increased from 567 members in 1982 to 1,606 members in 1992. A similar marked increase is seen in the membership figures of the Council for Acupuncture, from its earliest record of 510 members in 1984 to the 1992 level of 1,179 members. Some therapies, therefore, may be relatively short of practitioners with long clinical experience and so it may be beneficial to establish group practices to ensure a 'spread' of experience. Patients delegated by GPs to such 'centres of excellence' will have the benefit of a pool of professional experience which could be shared by a number of GP practices.[15] Another important consideration is that therapists are relatively few in number, particularly in certain parts of the country, and even one of the largest therapies such as osteopathy only has some 2,000 qualified practitioners. There might, therefore, be real benefits to the community if a number of GP practices were able to delegate the care of their patients to one or more local complementary-therapy practices.

Recent changes in the NHS have altered the context in which health care is delivered to patients. A national survey was undertaken in the autumn of 1992 by the University of Bradford

Clinical Epidemiology Research Unit, in conjunction with the National Association of Health Authorities and Trusts (NAHAT). Questionnaires were sent to all district health authorities, FHSAs, and a sample of 200 GP fund-holders—the three sectors responsible for purchasing health care. The aim of the survey was to establish a national picture of purchasers' attitudes towards the availability of non-conventional therapy in the NHS and to explore current and future approaches to purchasing and funding such therapies. The therapies which were identified as the main focus of attention were acupuncture, osteopathy, chiropractic, homoeopathy, reflexology, and aromatherapy. Data will be available from this survey which should improve current knowledge of the demand and use of non-conventional therapy from different sources and the present means of funding such services. Useful background information on the factors affecting purchasing decisions and the type of contact between doctor and therapist should also be available.

4.4. Establishing levels of competence

The key issue in the delegation of care appears to be ascertaining the competence of the practitioner. Under Paragraph 28 of the latest NHS (General Medical Services) Regulations 1992, it is specified that in employing ancillary staff the doctor shall have regard, in particular, to '(a) that person's academic and vocational qualifications; and (b) that person's training and his experience in employment'.

Implicit in the discussion of standards of competence is the need for practitioners to be aware of the limits of competence; it is imperative that therapists do not treat individuals in cases which exceed their capacity, training, and competence. A parallel can be drawn with medically qualified practitioners, where the law requires that 'a doctor will possess a degree of skill and experience appropriate to the post he occupies and the tasks he undertakes'.[16]

Practitioners of non-conventional therapies, especially those of discrete clinical disciplines, should be trained to know the jurisdiction of their practice and its limitations. This is essential in order to prevent the application of inappropriate treatments, particularly in the case of the more interventive therapies. Therapists should know which conditions and individuals they will be unable to treat successfully and be able to identify when the patient should be directed to medically qualified practitioners.

Fundamental to the safeguarding of patient interests is the treatment of individuals by competent persons. Patients presenting directly to therapists and who have not previously seen their GP with the presenting problem should be encouraged to inform or, if they wish, allow the therapist to inform the GP that the patient is attending for treatment. The patient should also be encouraged to attend his or her GP for review at appropriate intervals. When a doctor refers or delegates care to a non-medically qualified therapist, it should be made clear to the patient that the therapist is not a doctor. The existing nomenclature can be confusing for the patient: for example, the term 'consultant podiatrist' gives the impression of medical status.

It is particularly important that therapists do not countermand instructions or prescriptions given by a doctor. One study by Murray and Shepherd (1988) cited the disturbing case of a hypertensive patient who had been 'instructed' by his homoeopath to request the GP to reduce the prescribed dosage of hypotensive drugs by one half.[17] This case illustrates the problems when conflicting advice is given by different sources.

The question of contra-indications to particular treatments or therapies should be the subject of explicit guidance from the regulatory body. There will be certain individuals presenting with symptoms or conditions which preclude absolutely treatment by a therapist. For instance, a massage therapist should be instantly alerted by an individual with signs which may be indicative of deep venous thrombosis. Recognition of contra-indications is an essential element in the establishing of competence of therapists, as failure to recognize such signs could result in injury to the individual patient. A list of absolute contra-indications for osteopathic treatment, for example, has been compiled by the General Council and Register of Osteopaths and is reproduced in Appendix 1.

It should be noted in discussing competence that certain skills of differential diagnosis are necessary for some therapists. The model outlined in the Kings Fund report on osteopathy states:

A practitioner must be trained to make an appropriate differential diagnosis based upon current knowledge of the basic medical sciences. This should include an awareness that pain associated with certain visceral disease can mimic pains originating from within the musculoskeletal system. It is essential therefore that a practitioner should be able to distinguish between pain of a biomechanical nature and that of visceral origin as well as determine whether a pain is derived from the site where it is experienced or referred from another part.[18]

While such skills are necessary for the competent practitioner, responsibility for a complete medical diagnosis rests with the doctor. For instance, the main non-conventional therapies should be aware of the signs and symptoms of cardiac insufficiency in patients and recognize that this may be a contra-indication to certain types of treatment and that the patient requires the attention of their registered medical practitioner. The exact medical diagnosis, however, would remain the province of the doctor. Conversely, medical practitioners would benefit from some knowledge of biomechanical and other processes in order that they may, if they choose, delegate appropriately to osteopaths and other non-conventional therapists. The key element for both the doctor and the therapist is understanding the different spheres of influence in which they operate. It is, therefore, necessary to consider actions which can be taken to improve communications and understanding between physicians and non-conventional practitioners in order to safeguard patients' health.

4.5. Understanding non-conventional therapies

Studies cited earlier indicate a persistent trend among doctors of a desire for more information on non-conventional therapies. For instance, the study by Reilly of GP trainees[19] showed that 81.4 per cent of the sample wished to train in one or more non-conventional therapy. However, it is important to distinguish here between training to practise and more general raising of awareness of basic principles and application of various techniques. The latter kind of training is likely to have a wider application for physicians, many of whom would find it impossible to devote the time required to provide non-conventional therapies themselves or who do not wish to do so. It may also be helpful for GPs and other doctors to be trained to identify appropriate cases to delegate to non-conventional therapists, although work-load and the pressure to keep abreast of trends in medical science may not allow busy doctors to take advantage of such courses. More research needs to be carried out to increase the precision of defining which patients may benefit from particular treatments.

While there are many competing claims on an overloaded undergraduate medical curriculum, one study of 592 medical students suggested that 69 per cent would like some form of education in non-conventional therapies, whether as discussion classes or practical training.[20] It has been suggested (in Reilly's study, cited above) that some form of study of non-conventional therapies is useful, not simply because doctors will regularly encounter patients who have used such therapies, but also because the process of examining how to validate different techniques can be a very useful means of discussing scientific method and the nature of scientific proof with students.

Foundation courses on the methods and principles of key non-conventional therapies should be available to medical practitioners. This can be given to doctors in training or under continuing education arrangements for qualified doctors. Provision exists under section 63 of the Health Services and Public Health Act 1968 for trainee doctors to receive 'such instruction . . . as appears conducive to securing their efficiency [as practitioners]'. In addition, postgraduate education allowance (PGEA) approval for training qualified general practitioners may be granted by the Regional Adviser for General Practice, providing that such courses demonstrate 'acceptable educational content'. Medical practitioners seeking reimbursement for seminars or courses in aspects of non-conventional therapies should approach their regional adviser; a full list is given in Appendix 2.

Doctors need to know more about non-conventional therapies, not only for appropriate delegation of care, but also in their role as trusted adviser to their patients. As has been stated, doctors have a 'professional obligation to their patients to help guide them through the claims and counterclaims of practitioners on the medical fringe'.[21] General practitioners and other doctors coming into regular contact with patients are often asked for advice as to particular treatments and therapies on offer. The study of GPs in Oxfordshire cited earlier showed that 95 per cent of the sample had been approached by patients in the past year for information and advice on some form of non-conventional therapy.

Members of the public also need to be better informed about the non-conventional therapies which they use so that they can be discerning consumers; results of a Gallup poll of 978 people commissioned by the British Chiropractic Association revealed that 70 per cent of those surveyed did not know what area of the body was treated by a chiropractor (7 per cent believing it to be the feet).[22]

In order that doctors may be able to offer constructive advice when the patient makes enquiries about different techniques, it may be helpful for general practitioners to acquaint themselves with the local provision of non-conventional therapies. In order to foster greater understanding, therapists could hold 'open days' for GPs and other interested health-care professionals in order to demonstrate the services and standards of care on offer. It is through this kind of informal contact that greater mutual understanding can be achieved, which can only be to the benefit of patients.

At present, doctors do not always ask patients during consultations whether they have received some form of non-conventional treatment. Such information may be important, for instance if the treatment is in the form of a medicinal product which reacts in some way with prescribed medication. Doctors should, therefore, ask patients about their use of non-conventional therapies whenever they obtain a medical history.

A study by Budd and colleagues in 1990 piloted one model of integration of non-complementary therapies within the primary health-care setting.[23] This experiment, in which osteopathy and acupuncture were offered free of charge to patients at an NHS general practice in south London, highlighted important legal and ethical implications. The issues raised included access to patient records and the attendant questions of confidentiality, as well as practical concerns regarding insurance, sharing of practice prem- ises, and the like. It is important that these issues should be discussed by the appropriate bodies and resolved, where possible; forthcoming guidance in the form of a new edition of the Handbook of Medical Ethics will shortly be available from the BMA.[24]

Innovative multi-sectoral centres of investigation into aspects of non-conventional therapy include the Centre for Complementary Health Studies in Exeter, the Centre for the Study of Complemen- tary Medicine in Southampton and the Marylebone Centre Trust. A recent article based on the experience of the latter outlines some of the strengths and the problems associated with such multidis- ciplinary practices.[25] One experimental model of postgraduate education was developed with the Faculty of Homoeopathy to answer the question: 'Can general practitioners integrate selected elements of a complementary therapy in NHS practice?' Medical practitioners were given information and training in order to evaluate the claims made by a therapy and their resulting clinical behaviour was audited.

Collaboration between conventional and non-conventional prac- titioners has been important in improving mutual understanding and also in furthering our understanding of the value of different therapies. Criticism of many non-conventional therapies has focused on the paucity of sound scientific scrutiny of different techniques. In considering the relationship between the medical community and non-conventional therapists, it is worth reviewing in a little more detail the process of scientific evaluation of forms of health care.

4.6. Collaboration and research

Research is important in any field of medicine for several reasons. First, research is an important method of validation for a particular treatment or therapy; the rigorous testing of hypotheses is the hallmark of a sound science. Secondly, research is a valuable method of communication between fellow practitioners and a way of developing professional links within a given discipline.

Practitioners of orthodox medicine and non-conventional therapies should be prepared to conduct or arrange for research into their methods and practice. Two assertions sometimes made about non-conventional therapies and research need to be challenged. One is that these techniques are self-evidently effective and so their evaluation in trials where some patients would receive other treatments would be unethical. Time has shown that the occasions on which formal assessments are unnecessary are rare, and even in these exceptional circumstances research is still necessary to determine the most effective method of their use.

In addition, the true value of any treatment depends not only on its benefits but also its hazards, and here the unexpected but real retinal damage resulting from oxygen therapy in premature babies is cautionary.[27] The high oxygen concentrations that were often routinely used in the early 1950s almost certainly caused several thousand cases of retinopathy of prematurity (ROP), although it was not until the question had been investigated through trials that the hazard of ROP was clearly indicated. It was subsequently suggested that, although oxygen restriction had reduced ROP, mortality might have increased because some infants with respiratory-distress syndrome needed more oxygen than they received. This conclusion, however, which was not based on the results of investigative trials, has been challenged. The optimal approach, whenever possible, is to investigate not only the benefits but also the different hazards in the same trial(s).

Results from trials may confound expectations and assumptions previously held by experienced practitioners. Peckham cites the example from the Medical Research Council trial on the use of chorion villus sampling to detect genetic and cytogenetic disorders of the foetus in the first trimester of pregnancy.[28] Initially a randomized trial against amniocentesis in the second trimester was resisted, since chorion villus sampling had the advantage of earlier diagnosis. However, the results of the trial showed that chorion villus sampling differed from amniocentesis in terms of safety, accuracy, and the need for further testing. This example illustrates the importance of subjecting even 'self-evidently' beneficial therapies to rigorous testing and investigation.

The second assertion sometimes mounted against the testing of non-conventional therapies by established scientific means is that these therapies are so different from conventional methods that they cannot be investigated through clinical trials. However, all techniques, whether non-conventional or orthodox, aim to achieve particular objectives, which can be measured, even if this is easier for some than others. The Research Council for Complementary Medicine (RCCM) has highlighted this point in its submission to the COST project, outlined at the end of Chapter 2. This draft proposal states:

Proponents of unconventional medicine claim that they need specific methods of scientific evaluation which cannot necessarily be satisfied by the existing research routines. While this is certainly the case in some instances, the representatives of conventional medicine are probably correct in maintaining that quite often the existing scientific methods and criteria of efficacy could very well and meaningfully be applied to the evaluation of unconventional medicine.[29]

The advantages of randomized clinical trials, whereby subjects are allocated at random to the experimental treatment, such as a particular drug therapy, and a control regimen are well documented. The benefits of both the subject and the researcher being unaware of which regimen is being followed—a 'double-blind' trial—has also been demonstrated. The first double-blind individual randomization trial was carried out in 1948 in the MRC investigation into streptomycin,[30] seventeen years after the first group randomization trial in the US. Almost half-a-century of experience indicates that non-conventional therapies could benefit from the appropriate use of this method, alongside other established methods of scientific research. While difficulties of time, expense, and the considerable ethical problems[31] of randomization and informed consent should not be minimized, Professor Peckham, Director of Research and Development at the NHS, maintains that 'a randomized trial remains the best way of assessing whether a medical hunch is correct or incorrect'.[32] He believes that a 'stepwise' approach to assessment is required, using a combination of methods such as historical controls, case-control studies, and non-randomized current controls with adjustment techniques, culminating in the use of randomized controlled trials.

It should be noted in this respect that some illnesses may be self-limiting; patients suffering from conditions such as multiple sclerosis, for example, may experience episodes of spontaneous remission. It is important to attempt to distinguish the natural course of the disease which may be self-limiting from the effects of any intervention; it is only by carefully designed research that the effect of the treatment itself can be monitored. In addition, there will be individual variation to any treatment, whether conventional or non-conventional; research studies should help to establish the range of that variation.

The question of efficacy—how to judge the ability of a treatment to produce the intended result—is clearly a difficult one. Much debate has been generated recently regarding the measurement of *outcomes* of treatment. Self-reported general health status or quality-of-life measures are used increasingly in research in orthodox medicine,[33] using protocols such as the Nottingham Health Profile. These developments are useful in reminding us that it may not always be appropriate to think of efficacy in terms only of relieving a sign or symptom. Such measures may play a useful part in developing sensitive research instruments for non-conventional therapies.

Research to compare the effectiveness and safety of non-conventional therapies either with conventional techniques or with other non-conventional methods is best carried out through randomized treatment comparisons. The purpose of allocating treatments at random within the eligible study population is to establish identical, or at least very similar, groups so that treatment is the only variable that could account for any difference observed between the groups at the end of the study. This approach is more feasible than has so far been generally recognized. The results of such trials will inform professional groups, both orthodox and non-conventional, about the value of different approaches. They will also enable patients to make rational decisions so that they can take advantage of methods that are effective.

The resources needed to evaluate clinical practice to the highest standard, whether in orthodox or non-conventional treatment, are considerable. Non-conventional therapists may lack the time, money, experience, and infrastructure to carry out research trials. It has been noted that: 'There is a clamour for more research in complementary medicine but, at the same time, there is a dearth of resources and of experienced individuals to take on the work.'[34] The advent of degree courses for certain non-conventional disciplines should encourage the development of a research ethos into the main therapies.

The organizational structure of medical research is well established, with the dual support mechanism of the Universities Funding Council and the research councils; the academic discipline of investigation into non-conventional therapies is more embryonic in universities and research establishments. The financial support of the pharmaceutical industry is also a factor in the healthy state of orthodox medical science; it was estimated by the House of Lords Select Committee on Science and Technology that the pharmaceutical industry was the source of 66.3 per cent of all funding for medical research.[35] Research into non-conventional therapies are highly unlikely to attract similar financial support. It has also been noted that there is a lack of an equivalent in non-conventional therapies to the registrar grade in medical schools, whose job specification includes the implementation of research projects under the experienced guidance of their professional mentors.[36]

It is for these reasons that advice and support given by organizations such as the Research Council for Complementary Medicine (RCCM) is so valuable. (Equally welcome is the development of research agencies for single therapies such as the Homoeopathic Medical Research Council. It is likely that other therapies may establish their own research bodies, specific to those therapies, in future years. In the meantime, the existence of an 'umbrella' research body such as the RCCM is welcome.) The RCCM was set up as an independent charity in 1983 and performs a valuable service in providing advice, funding, and support for research in different therapies. It has also worked with the British Library to develop impressive information resources in non-conventional therapies, including a computerized database of abstracts and other research data. One important function of the RCCM is to provide advice as to research methodology—for instance, the setting up of clinical trials—and to assist individual researchers in producing appropriate research protocols. Such moves are an encouraging sign of the willingness of different therapies to subject themselves to rigorous evaluation and independent scrutiny.

It is recognized that some of the criticisms levelled against non-conventional therapies in terms of poor information on outcomes and effectiveness of treatment, would also hold true for certain areas of orthodox medicine.[37] For instance, Fisher and colleagues have noted in one example that: 'The mode of action of penicillinamine in rheumatoid arthritis is unknown but it is a valuable treatment.'[38] One welcome new initiative to provide more information on existing evidence relating to the effectiveness of different treatments is the Cochrane Centre. This was set up in 1992 by the NHS Research and Development Division as a central clearing-house for clinical trials, and represents a positive step forward in consolidating current health research.

Training in the 'building blocks' of research methodology should feature as part of the undergraduate curriculum for the discrete clinical disciplines (see Chapter 5). This could include components of survey design and execution, presenting and analysing data, statistics, and information technology. Very simple retrospective research projects could be undertaken within the therapist's own practice to establish a base-line of knowledge within each therapy, such as the demographics and presenting problems of patients. Some general books which may be helpful for the individual therapist or medical practitioner wishing to undertake or participate in research in non-conventional treatment methods are listed in Appendix 3.

An important initiative to foster greater collaboration between medical science and non-conventional therapies is the Fellowship in Research Methodology which was established conjointly by the

Research Council for Complementary Medicine, the Medical Research Council, and the University of Glasgow. The preliminary results of this investigation,[39] which considered the use of established scientific methods of evaluation for non-conventional therapies, should stimulate debate on methods of constructive collaboration between orthodox medicine and non-conventional therapies. More detailed information on recent developments in research in different therapies is given in Chapter 7.

Another welcome development in furthering existing knowledge is the establishment of a database into adverse effects of different non-conventional medicines at the National Poisons Unit.[40] This surveillance scheme combines the recording of events with the *validation* of data by on-site clinical toxicologists; this enables cases to be confirmed by specialists before being entered in the database. This project is currently receiving joint funding from the Ministry of Agriculture, Fisheries, and Food and the Department of Health. The necessity for such a monitoring system is indicated by the fact that few herbal medicines have been through any form of rigorous drug trial, although under forthcoming EC legislation, discussed in Chapter 2, such products may soon be subject to stricter controls.

When considering possible adverse effects of herbal and other medicines, an important area for further research is a consideration of the consequences of *combining* different therapeutic treatments on a patient. It is not known yet whether one treatment cancels out another or what are the effects on the patient in terms of possible fragmentation of care. This area could usefully be the subject of further monitoring and research.

Although the evaluation of different techniques is the most obvious application of research into non-conventional therapies, there are of course other reasons for encouraging it. These include the aim—as an end in itself—of inculcating critical awareness among the practitioners. In addition, surveys and other simple research tolls may be useful in establishing the prevalence and incidence of conditions for which non-conventional methods may be useful and the monitoring of changes in these indices over time. The dearth of basic data on the number of practising therapists and the methods of treatment on offer has already been noted.

Simple research on work-load and patient demographics could be undertaken by practitioners, as part of a research and auditing programme. As Professor Ginsburg has stated: 'Complementary practitioners must be prepared to change what they do in the light of research findings and to participate in the processes of inquiry.'[41] Registration on a therapy-by-therapy basis should result in more accurate information on the scope and nature of different therapies. More generally, a commitment to research and to the dissemination of results provides a valuable method of communication between fellow practitioners.

4.7. Summary

Doctors have always had discretion to transfer portions of patient care to non-medical practitioners; these powers have become wider in recent times. In these circumstances, the doctor retains clinical responsibility for the patient during the time of treatment by a designated practitioner, such as a chiropodist or osteopath. It is, therefore, imperative that practitioners should be able to prove that they have attained recognized levels of competence in that field, so that the doctor may have confidence in making arrangements with a therapist for the care of a patient. Defined levels of competence should be set for each therapy to guide the doctor and to safeguard the patient against unskilled or unqualified practitioners.

It is not known how many doctors practise some form of non-conventional therapy, as estimates range from about 2 per cent to over 15 per cent. Doctors practising non-conventional therapies remain accountable to the General Medical Council for whatever treatment they administer to the patient. However, where there are clear and recognized standards of competence laid down for a given therapy, these should be observed by all therapists, whether medically qualified or not.

Seminars and courses on the principles and methods of key therapies should be available to medical practitioners. Increased understanding of such techniques enables doctors to delegate care appropriately and advise patients about the benefits and hazards of different treatments. Provision exists for vocational training in such therapies and for postgraduate education allowances; medical practitioners wishing to undertake such training should seek the guidance of their regional adviser.

Closer collaboration between the medical profession and practitioners of non-conventional medicine in clinical research should be encouraged. In particular, active support is needed for therapists embarking on research, both in terms of funding and appropriate training. The dearth of information on patient consultations with therapists would make simple research into work-load and case-mix helpful. Registering bodies should ensure that members keep records to enable such monitoring to be undertaken.

5 *The regulation debate*

5.1. Regulation—a risk-assessment model

The control of non-conventional therapies has long been a subject of intense debate in parliament and in professional and public arenas. Recent years have seen important developments in the self-regulation of different therapies and some encouraging initiatives to raise standards in non-conventional treatments. Before reviewing the results of the BMA survey detailing the activities of non-conventional therapists and their representative bodies, it is necessary to consider briefly in this chapter the issues surrounding the regulation of such therapies and to sketch out possible future developments.

The value of any treatment depends on the balance between the likely benefits and harms, since it cannot be assumed that any given therapy or method of medical practice is completely harmless. When considering non-conventional therapies, the most innocuous of practices may be harmful if they prevent the patient from seeking other, more appropriate treatment. In the case of a patient with a surgically amenable cancer presenting to a non-conventional therapist, delay in being seen by a doctor would be a matter of concern if during that time the cancer metastasized and a successful outcome from surgery became less likely.

It is important to make the distinction between those therapies which at worst will have a placebo effect but may cause patients to delay seeking appropriate treatment, and those methods which in themselves could be harmful in the hands of an unskilled practitioner. Therapies such as acupuncture, osteopathy, and chiropractic clearly have the potential to do harm as well as good because they involve physical manipulation or invasive techniques. In this way they cannot be considered in the same light as adjunctive therapies such as healing or Bach flower remedies, which are most unlikely to be harmful in themselves.

Because of the diverse nature of those methods loosely grouped together as non-conventional therapies, different categories should be established. Such a taxonomy is important in order to distinguish between those therapies which require rigorous training similar to an undergraduate medical course and those which can be taught adequately in short courses or seminars. The distinctions are also important in terms of the different systems of control which are appropriate for these different methods. Pietroni has devised the following categories,[1] with examples of treatments for each distinct area given below:

Complete systems
Homoeopathy, osteopathy, herbal medicine, acupuncture

Diagnostic methods
Iridology, kinesiology, hair analysis

Therapeutic modalities
Massage, shiatsu, reflexology

Self-care approaches
Meditation, yoga, relaxation

5.2. Discrete clinical disciplines

This taxonomy would appear to make sense in terms of discriminating between therapies which in their aspirations and practice are so very different. It is perhaps the first tier which is of most interest to this report, for two reasons. First, the four therapies listed above in Pietroni's schemata (osteopathy, acupuncture, homoeopathy, and herbalism) together with chiropractic make up the most common therapies used in the UK today according to the Consumers Association. Secondly, these therapies probably have the greatest potential to do harm to the patient.

Pietroni labelled this category as 'complete systems', although it is arguable whether a therapy such as osteopathy claims to be a whole system of medicine. These therapies could perhaps better be named *discrete clinical disciplines*. They are distinguished from other therapies by having more established foundations of training and have, to differing degrees, established criteria of competence and professional standards. Within defined parameters, these therapies perhaps have the greatest potential for use in conjunction with orthodox structures of health care.

It is clear that discrete clinical disciplines, as defined above, and self-care approaches will have very different educational and regulatory needs. Other therapies fall between these two poles, for instance, hypnotherapy may be used as a technique for a specific condition (pain relief during tooth extraction) or for more general psychotherapeutic uses; it is clear that there may be greater risks associated with different *uses* of a therapy, as well as for different therapies. Recognition of these differences informs decisions about which therapies should be subject to regulation by statute and which can be satisfactorily controlled by voluntary regulation procedures alone.

5.3.   Statutory versus voluntary regulation

It should be noted that no single method of control will be suitable for all forms of non-conventional therapy. Those therapies posing greater potential risks to patients require *legal regulation by statute* to protect consumers from unskilled or incompetent practitioners. The UK government has openly welcomed the progress which has been made by some of the non-conventional therapies in developing credible systems of self-regulation. There also appears to be recognition that self-regulation in some circumstances will probably require the force of law. Before any therapy can be considered for statutory regulation, the government believes that certain criteria would have to be fulfilled. The following conditions have been laid down by the government for any therapy seeking statutory regulation:[2]

that the therapy has been long established and has an established and credible system of voluntary regulation;

that there should be recognized courses of training, including a structured system of assessment with external examiners;

that there is consensus upon the way forward amongst all the different organizations within that therapy;

that the medical profession is broadly supportive of the move towards statutory regulation.

It can be seen that those therapies which have been categorized here as discrete clinical disciplines are probably the most suitable candidates for statutory regulation, as indicated by the government criteria above. In addition to these four pre-conditions should be added the question of relative risk or the potential to harm the patient. This makes control of discrete clinical disciplines more pressing than that of non-interventive techniques.

A special caveat should be attached to the regulation of herbalism and homoeopathy. As mentioned in Chapter 2, existing medicines regulation is likely to be extended to cover the marketing and dispensing of 'natural' and homoeopathic medicinal products. This legislation, emanating from Brussels, is likely to provide sufficient regulatory controls for the consumer in these areas; however, such therapies, because of their potential to do harm, should follow best practice as outlined in the next chapter.

In reviewing recent developments in regulation among the different non-conventional therapies, it is worth considering briefly the model of statutory regulation for osteopaths. The process by which recognition was achieved for osteopaths illustrates the importance of the criteria for statutory regulation set out above. The regulation of osteopathy may well provide a useful model for other therapies which reach a similar stage of development.

5.4. Osteopathy—a case study

Osteopathy is the first therapy to put forward a system of statutory regulation, and this has been welcomed by the British Medical Association and other leading bodies. Until recently there were

eight distinct osteopathic organizations with a registering function—later streamlined to five—and it is to the credit of the
osteopathic profession that consensus was achieved in drawing up
this exemplary model of regulation.

Attempts to regulate osteopathy have been on the statute books
for some sixty years. In the space of one period of just five years,
three separate bills seeking to regulate osteopathy were presented
to Parliament in 1931, 1933, and 1934. The BMA produced
evidence in 1935 to the House of Lords Select Committee
considering a Registration Bill on osteopathy which was later
withdrawn. The BMA evidence was critical of the wider claims of
the discipline, while recognizing 'manipulation as a valuable
method of treatment in certain conditions'.[3] Study of the earlier
abortive attempts of the osteopaths to achieve statutory regulation[4] is instructive as an illustration of the real difficulties which
had to be surmounted in the preparation of the present model.

In 1991 a working-party of the Kings Fund (King Edward's
Hospital Fund for London) produced a report which recommended that osteopathy should be subject to a system of statutory
registration which would include a restriction of the title 'osteopath'. The working-party proposed that a General Osteopathic
Council should be established to regulate the practice of the
profession of osteopathy by establishing and maintaining minimum standards of training and enforcing an appropriate code of
professional conduct. Following on from the Kings Fund report, a
bill to regulate the profession of osteopathy was introduced into
the House of Lords in the summer of 1991 by Lord Walton, a past
president of the BMA and the General Medical Council. The bill
attracted all-party and government support but fell in March
1992 after completing its committee stage when Parliament was
dissolved prior to the general election. The bill provided for the
regulation of all established osteopathic practitioners and the
restriction of the title 'osteopathy'. A second reading took place in
the House of Commons on 15 January 1993, and the bill is now
passing through committee stages. When enacted, this legislation
will not prevent practitioners such as physiotherapists and

manipulative therapists from carrying out manual or manipulative forms of treatment. A similar working-party investigation is currently being undertaken by the Kings Fund into the regulation of chiropractic.

In discussing the regulation of non-conventional therapies, it is worth considering two questions which recur in debate on the subject. The first is the notion of a single over-arching regulatory body covering the whole spectrum of therapies. This is discussed below, followed by a brief consideration of the feasibility of extending the Council for the Professions Supplementary to Medicine to encompass different non-conventional therapies.

5.5. Umbrella bodies

The possibility of establishing a single regulatory structure governing all non-conventional therapies has often been discussed; indeed, there are at present a panoply of such organizations claiming to represent a wide range of therapies. While these organizations have attempted to formulate common codes of conduct and standards within some of the less well-known non-conventional therapies, it appears that the concept of a single umbrella group is no longer seen as an effective way forward for the regulation of non-conventional therapies. Indeed, the government's change of stance on this matter was made explicit in the debate in the House of Lords in May 1990; given the importance of this policy development, it is perhaps worth reproducing the comments of Baroness Hooper in full. She stated at the beginning of the debate that:

The Government's stance on umbrella bodies has changed in recent years. There is little homogeneity among the various natural therapy professions, and the major groups now see their way forward not through umbrella organisations but by a group by group approach following consensus within their ranks. After all, if we look at orthodox medicine for a model we see for example that the medical and dental practitioners, clinical psychologists and ophthalmologists have far more in common with one another than the vast majority of natural therapists, yet they all have independent and individual governing and registering bodies and associations which represent their interests.

At one time, we were of the view that there might be advantages if all the natural therapies came together in mutual understanding. But, given the diversity, practice and aspirations of those professions—coupled perhaps with their increasing proliferation—we now believe very firmly that it must be for each therapy group to determine its own future development.[5]

5.6. Professions supplementary to medicine

In considering the relationship between different sectors of health care, analogies are sometimes made between non-conventional therapists and the diverse groups loosely banded together as 'professions supplementary to medicine'. It is sometimes suggested that one or other of the non-conventional therapies could be added to the seven currently regulated by the Council for Professions Supplementary to Medicine, each of which has its own code of practice and conduct.

The Professions Supplementary to Medicine Act 1960 requires that physiotherapists, chiropodists, dietitians, medical laboratory scientific officers, occupational therapists, radiographers, and orthoptists who work in the NHS or for the personal social-service departments of local authorities must satisfy defined minimum levels of training. In addition, there is an obligation for these individuals to register with the Council for Professions Supplementary to Medicine (CPSM). However, practitioners who work in the private sector are not legally obliged to register with the CPSM. In addition, any training body wishing to train students solely for private practice need not apply for CPSM approval.

The limitations of the CPSM are considerable, given the high proportion of individuals in these various professions working outside the NHS or local authorities. It is estimated that there are as many physiotherapists in full-time private practice as there are those in NHS or local-authority employment. It can be seen that neither the CPSM nor its professional boards has any effective control over professionals working solely in the private sector. It should be noted that in the private sector it can often be difficult to establish the credentials even of doctors. This would be more true of non-conventional therapies, even where therapies are subject to registration. Given that most non-conventional therapists at present are private practitioners, it is unlikely that the addition of various therapies to the current range of professions under the auspices of the CPSM would provide satisfactory solutions in terms of the regulation of these therapies. Such arrangements would therefore be inadequate in protecting the public from possible harm.

5.7.   Summary

The individual seeking the help of a non-conventional therapist should ask the following questions:

- Is the therapist registered with a professional oganization?
- Does this body have a:
  —public register;
  —code of practice;
  —effective disciplinary procedure and sanctions;
  —complaints mechanism?
- What qualifications does the therapist hold? What type/ length/quality of training has been undertaken to obtain these qualifications?
- How many years has the therapist been practising?
- Is the therapist covered by professional indemnity insurance?

Not all non-conventional therapies require regulation by statute. For the majority of therapies, adoption of a code of practice, training structures, and voluntary registration would be sufficient. The discrete clinical disciplines of osteopathy, chiropractic, acupuncture, homoeopathy, and herbalism should be subject to regulation by statute in forthcoming years. This applies in particular to the manipulative therapies (osteopathy, chiropractic) and acupuncture, on the grounds that their continuing unregulated practice poses a potential danger to patients. It may well be considered that existing and future legislation in the UK and Europe on herbal and homoeopathic medicines will be sufficient to regulate the therapies of homoeopathy and herbal medicine.

What is certain, however, is that if some of the non-conventional therapies are regulated by statute, such measures will simply be an exercise in statutory self-registration and will not imply 'recognition' of a particular therapy or provide for its inclusion within the National Health Service.

6 *BMA survey of non-conventional therapies*

6.1. Survey method

There are currently very few data on the practice and control of non-conventional therapies in the UK. The exact number of practising therapies in the UK has not been confirmed, nor a precise tally given of the membership of different organizations associated with various therapies. The panoply of bodies claiming to represent different practices can be very confusing even to the most discerning of consumers. The British Medical Association Board of Science and Education, in an attempt to elucidate present patterns of use and organization of different therapies, conducted a national survey of non-conventional therapies in 1991. A detailed questionnaire was sent out with questions on the organization, practice, training, qualifications, and research for a wide range of therapies. The original questionnaire is given for information in Appendix 4.

The principal therapies used in the UK today have been identified by the Consumers Association[1] as osteopathy, chiropractic, homoeopathy, acupuncture, and herbalism. Other therapies widely used include aromatherapy, reflexology, and hypnotherapy. The bodies representing these major therapies were approached by the BMA, together with organizations representing other therapies, including Bach flower remedies, healing, iridology, and massage. Appropriate bodies were identified initially by use of two key source-books: Fulder's 1988 *Handbook of Complementary Medicine* and the 1990 *Natural Medicine Practitioners' Yearbook*.[2]

It should be noted that the survey was not intended as a comprehensive census. As has been noted before, 160 different therapies and their offshoots were identified by one observer, and it would not be practicable to approach each and every organization in existence. It is, however, likely that the main therapies currently available in the UK are represented in this survey.

It was decided that organizations consisting solely of medical membership would be excluded, as the control mechanisms for individuals was already established by membership of the General Medical Council. The exception to this was the Faculty of Homoeopathy which was approached for the reason that homoeopathy has a special relationship to the National Health Service. However, it was chiefly the 'lay' groups which were targeted for response, as the main objective of the survey was to identify the channels of control and representation within different therapies.

Also outside the remit of this survey were the 'umbrella' groups which claim to represent more than one therapy. The detailed information on training, research, practice, and control which we wished to obtain for each therapy surveyed would not necessarily be available from such general bodies. In addition, the inclusion of umbrella bodies may have resulted in unnecessary and confusing duplication of material. The question of 'umbrella' bodies and the different mechanisms by which therapies can be regulated were discussed in the previous chapter. There appears to be a general drift among therapists, parliamentarians, and others away from umbrella bodies towards single registering bodies for each therapy. For this reason, organizations representing more than one therapy—umbrella bodies—were not included in this survey.

Forty organizations representing a range of therapies were sent a letter explaining the purpose of the survey and a copy of the questionnaire. Three organizations were not contactable at the given addresses and so were excluded from the survey; in addition, one body did not wish to participate in the survey. Completed questionnaires were received from twenty-seven organizations including one organization that was also answering for another. These twenty-seven responses covered acupuncture, Alexander technique, aromatherapy, Bach flower remedies, chiropractic, crystal healing, healing, herbalism, homoeopathy, hypnotherapy, iridology, kinesiology, massage, osteopathy, radionics, reflexology, and shiatsu. The difference between the twenty-eight replies and the seventeen therapies is accounted for by some of the therapies having more than one parent organization.

Having received the questionnaires, together with accompanying evidence in the form of course curricula, prospectuses, codes of ethics and practice, and other written material, the data were summarized in tabular form. This summary of information provided by each organization was then returned to each originating body to be checked, and individual organizations were given the opportunity to correct any errors or inaccuracies in the presentation before publication. The data provided by this exercise were not independently validated by the BMA or any other body.

The full results of the survey are given in the following section. While this information cannot be seen in any way as a guide or directory to all the different bodies currently in existence, it is hoped that the process of consultation with responding organizations has provided data which reflect the wide range and diversity of therapy groups whose practice falls generally within the scope of non-conventional therapies. The BMA would like to thank all organizations for their co-operation in responding to this survey.

6.2. Results

Responses to the BMA survey of non-conventional therapies were received from the following organizations:

Acupuncture	British Academy of Western Acupuncture; Council for Acupuncture
Alexander technique	Society of Teachers of the Alexander Technique
Aromatherapy	International Federation of Aromatherapists; Register of Qualified Aromatherapists
Bach flower remedies	Dr Edward Bach Centre
Chiropractic	British Chiropractic Association
Crystal healing	International Association of Crystal Healing Therapists
Healing	Aetherius Society; Confederation of Healing Organizations
Herbalism	General Council and Register of Consultant Herbalists; National Institute of Medical Herbalists
Homoeopathy	Faculty of Homoeopathy; Society of Homoeopaths
Hypnotherapy	National Council of Psychotherapists and Hypnotherapy Register
Iridology	British Society of Iridologists
Kinesiology	Association for Systematic Kinesiology
Massage	London College of Massage
Osteopathy	College of Osteopaths Practitioners Association; General Council and Register of Osteopaths; Natural Therapeutic and Osteopathic Society and Register
Radionics	British Biomagnetics Association; Confederation of Radionics and Radiesthetic

	Organizations; Institute of Signalysis Practitioners
Reflexology	Association of Reflexologists; British Reflexology Association
Shiatsu	Shiatsu Society

Summaries were prepared from the responses received and were sent for confirmation to the responding organizations. These approved summaries are reproduced on the following pages, for the information of the reader. These are presented in the order given above, by main therapy group listed alphabetically.

TABLE 6.1 **British Academy of Western Acupuncture** (n = 190)

Section One: *Organization*

Functions of organization	Details — Number of staff	Council/committee structure	Premises	Company status	Register of members
To promote the availability of acupuncture to patients in the West.	Part-time voluntary (no numbers).	Board of Governors, elected at the AGM (all members invited).	No permanent premises.	Charitable organization.	Yes.

Section Two: *Practice*

Conditions treated	Methods	Patient's GP informed of treatment?	Referral by GP	Concurrent treatment	Ethical code
Wide range including: nervous tension, asthma, bronchitis, arthritis, Bell's palsy, cystitis, skin conditions, PMT, dysmenorrhoea, hay fever, migraine, depression, enuresis, sciatica.	Needles with or without moxibustion and electropuncture.	Usually, but not a requirement for members to inform GP.	Yes in pain clinics; otherwise no.	Yes. Independent of orthodox therapy.	Yes.

Section Three: *Training and qualification*

Entry qualifications	Clinical training	Post-graduate training	Examination	Course duration	Qualification	Course approval	Medical input in training
2 years postgraduate study. Physiotherapists, registered nurses or doctors.	Students practise on each other.	Annual training course.	Multiple choice; essay, practical. No external monitoring. Structured working.	2 months i.e. 8 weekends. 12 hours/weekend.	Passing the exam at end of course.	Approved by board of governors.	President. 2 course tutors are GPs.

Section Four: *Research*

Research by organization	Research by another organization	Commissioned research	References in peer-reviewed journal	Own journal
No.	No.	No.	No—argues that use traditional acupuncture points as adjunct to established western medicine.	Yes (newsletter).

TABLE 6.2 Council for Acupuncture (CFA) (n =1,114)

Section One: *Organization*

Functions of organization	Details		Premises	Company status	Register of members
	Number of staff	Council/committee structure			
Act as forum for member bodies of Council to recommend standards of education, training, qualification, ethics, and discipline. To seek statutory registration for member bodies of the Council 'who may be desirous' of such registration.	1 part-time secretary for CFA itself. Each member body employs a secretary/registrar.	Governing Council elected at annual meetings.	Registered office.	Limited company.	Yes. Each member body holds a register and Council keeps overall directory.

Section Two: *Practice*

Conditions treated	Methods	Patient's GP informed of treatment?	Referral by GP	Concurrent treatment	Ethical code
Cite WHO 1979 list of conditions responsive to acupuncture, including diseases of the upper respiratory tract; respiratory system, gastro-intestinal system, eye and mouth; plus neurological and musculo-skeletal disorders.	Principally acupuncture, together with herbal medicines, dietary indications, and exercise regimens.	Usually, with consent of patient.	At times.	Yes.	Yes.

Section Three: *Training and qualification*

Entry qualifications	Clinical training	Post-graduate training	Examination	Course duration	Qualification	Course approval	Medical input in training
Equivalent to those required for tertiary education—5 GCSE 3 'A' levels.	Clinical instruction and assessment of clinical competence.	*Ad hoc* continuing education in the form of seminars, etc.	Written and practical.	Minimum two years full-time.	Different according to the professional body, e.g. MTAcS (Member of the Traditional Acupuncture Society).	Criteria laid down in the Handbook of British Acupuncture Accreditation Board.	None, but anatomy/physiology component of training.

Section Four: *Research*

Research by organization	Research by another organization	Commissioned research	References in peer-reviewed journal	Own journal
Yes—CFA has set up its own research sub-committee to review existing studies.	Yes—RCCM and others.	No (as yet).	Yes, numerous—e.g. *JAMA* 1975; 232; 1,133–5; or *J. Clin. Epidemiol.* 1990; 11: 1,191–9.	Yes—series of professional journals.

TABLE 6.3 Society of Teachers of the Alexander Technique (n = 846)

Section One: *Organization*

Functions of organization	Details		Council/committee structure	Premises	Company status	Register of members
	Number of staff					
Promoting teaching of Alexander Technique. Supervising standards of training. Maintaining and improving professional standards. Upholding the code of ethics dealing with infringements. Preventing exploitation by untrained people. Facilitating contact between the public and teachers. Facilitating contact between members. Encouraging research.	1 full-time administrator (paid). 1 part-time administrative assistant. 1 part-time office junior.		Council: Chairman, Treasurer, Secretary, and 6 Ordinary members elected at AGM. Sub-committees: Ethics, Industry, Medicine and Research, Publishing, Office administration and Trust Fund, Professional Development, Publicity, International Liaison, UK/EEC regulations.	Leased office.	Members' association.	Yes.

Section Two: *Practice*

Conditions treated	Methods	Patient's GP informed of treatment?	Referral by GP	Concurrent treatment	Ethical code
Can alleviate back pain, postural disorders, whiplash injury, breathing problems, myalgia rheumatica, RSI, hypertension, anxiety, stress, and other chronic conditions.	Teaching psycho-physical awareness, the basic principles and practice of poise and neuro-muscular co-ordination: how to change the habits of a lifetime.	Pupils with medical conditions usually advised to see GP.	Occasionally and increasingly.	Yes. Complementary to orthodox therapy.	Yes.

Section Three: *Training and qualification*

Entry qualifications	Clinical training	Post-graduate training	Examination	Course duration	Qualification	Course approval	Medical input in training
Good general education, mature personality. Interview. Sufficient previous Alexander experience.	Not appropriate.	Regular post-graduate and professional development courses.	Continuous practical and oral assessment. External moderation.	1600 hours (3 years), 80% practical.	Certificate.	By Society in London and by affiliated societies overseas.	Relevant Anatomy and Physiology.

Section Four: *Research*

Research by organization	Research by another organization	Commissioned research	References in peer-reviewed journal	Own journal
By individual members e.g. Barlow (1973). Jones (1979). Stevens (in press).	Individual Ph.D investigations in UK and US.	No.	Yes—*Ann.Phys. Med.* 1952; 1: 77–89. *Lancet* 1955; 659–64. *Psychol. Rev.* 1965; 72: 196–214. *Ann. Rev. Respir. Drs.* 1990; 141: A721.	Yes.

TABLE 6.4 International Federation of Aromatherapists (n = 1186)

Section One: *Organization*

Functions of organization	Details				Register of members
	Number of staff	Council/committee structure	Premises	Company status	
Governing and controlling body for the professional aromatherapist and source of information for the public.	Not given.	Elected council and subcommittees.	Office at Royal Masonic Hospital.	Registered charity.	Yes.

Section Two: *Practice*

Conditions treated	Methods	Patient's GP informed of treatment?	Referral by GP	Concurrent treatment	Ethical code
Stress and stress-related disorders.	Massage and essential oil application.	Yes, if appropriate.	Yes—estimated 28%	With the permission of GP or consultant.	Yes.

Section Three: *Training and qualification*

Entry qualifications	Clinical training	Post-graduate training	Examination	Course duration	Qualification	Course approval	Medical input in training
For full membership qualifications in anatomy, physiology, massage, and aromatherapy (none for ordinary membership).	Full-time minimum 300 hours. Part-time—depends on individual schools.	Advanced courses, workshops, etc.	Written, oral, and practical.	Full-time: min. 300 hours supervised training. Part-time: schools' own schedule.	Membership of IFA—looking towards NVQ.	IFA Education Examining Board.	Yes.

Section Four: *Research*

Research by organization	Research by another organization	Commissioned research	References in peer-reviewed journal	Own journal
Yes—cross-over trial in conjunction with the British Endometriosis Society.	Programme with the voluntary sector called 'Aromatherapy in Care'.	No.	No.	No.

TABLE 6.5 Register of Qualified Aromatherapists (n = 120)

Section One: *Organization*

Functions of organization	Details Number of staff	Council/committee structure	Premises	Company status	Register of members
1. To maintain high standards of professional training and practice in the field of aromatherapy, massage, and bodywork. 2. Forum for exchange of knowledge. 3. To promote public understanding of aromatherapy.	No paid staff (secretary paid an honorarium).	Executive Committee: Hon. Chairman, Presiding Chairman, Treasurer, Secretary, Training and Education Officer, Public Relations Officer, Research Officer.	No official leased premises— main office is home of secretary.	—	Yes.

Section Two: *Practice*

Conditions treated	Methods	Patient's GP informed of treatment?	Referral by GP	Concurrent treatment	Ethical code
Do not claim to 'treat' conditions like a GP, but may relieve stress-related problems, e.g. headaches, indigestion.	Massage with external use of plant essential oils (e.g. lavender) diluted in a base oil of vegetable origin.	Patients advised by therapists to inform GP, not usually by therapists direct.	Yes—occasionally.	Yes.	Yes.

Section Three: *Training and qualification*

Entry qualifications	Clinical training	Post-graduate training	Examination	Course duration	Qualification	Course approval	Medical input in training
None.	50 hours.	Seminars and postgraduate courses at the school.	Written, oral, and practical.	Minimum of 200 teaching contact hours, submission of 50 treatment reports, and a total of 300 hours of directed home study.	MRQA (Member of the Register of Qualified Aromatherapists).	Training Committee reviews syllabus; interviews Principal of School; and visits site for inspection.	Yes; teaching of anatomy, physiology, and biology of diseases.

Section Four: *Research*

Research by organization	Research by another organization	Commissioned research	References in peer-reviewed journal	Own journal
No.	Yes—but not available yet.	No.	No references given.	No.

TABLE 6.6 Dr Edward Bach Centre

Section One: *Organization*

Functions of organization	Details		Council/committee structure	Premises	Company status	Register of members
	Number of staff					
To promote Bach Flower Remedies (Private Ltd. Co. for preparation of products at same offices). Foundation for teaching and conducting courses in the use of Bach Flower Remedies.	Six.		3 Trustees of Dr E. Bach Trust. 3 Directors of Edward Bach Foundation. 3 Directors of BFR (Mount Vernon) Ltd.	Registered offices for the Edward Bach Foundation and BFR (Mount Vernon) Ltd.	Private Limited company for preparation of the remedies; also a Charitable Trust at same premises.	No.

Section Two: *Practice*

Conditions treated	Methods	Patient's GP informed of treatment?	Referral by GP	Concurrent treatment	Ethical code
Negative emotional outlooks.	Flowers from wild plants, bushes, and trees.	Patients usually advised to inform GP themselves.	Occasionally.	Yes.	Yes. In accordance with Dr Bach's teachings.

Section Three: *Training and qualification*

Entry qualifications	Clinical training	Post-graduate training	Examination	Course duration	Qualification	Course approval	Medical input in training
None.	3 days at Bach Centre. 3 months correspondence 'practical' course.	Annual review.	Written assessment and essay paper in Part I. Three case studies and 1 essay in Part II. Monitoring by correspondence and appraisal.	17 hours at Bach Centre. Practical correspondence course.	Successful students entered on Register.	Approved by registered offices.	Course conducted by 2 registered nurses.

Section Four: *Research*

Research by organization	Research by another organization	Commissioned research	References in peer-reviewed journal	Own journal
Yes—research finalized by founder Dr Edward Bach.	No.	No.	No.	Yes (newsletter).

TABLE 6.7 British Chiropractic Association (n = 450)

Section One: *Organization*

Functions of organization	Details		Council/committee structure	Premises	Company status	Register of members
	Number of staff					
To campaign for statutory legislation for the chiropractic profession in the UK. To enforce code of ethics and practice for members. Encourage research and development into chiropractic procedures. Promotion of the chiropractic profession.	1 full-time office administrator. 2 part-time Parliamentary Officers, Communications Officer. 4 part-time on contract, including Marketing Consultant and X-ray Standards and Radiation Protection Adviser.		Council: Assistant Secretary and 4 Council members (elected at AGM). Day-to-day running of the Assoc. by Finance and General Purposes Committee, consisting of President, Vice-President, Treasurer and Secretary. Council directs 22 committees, e.g. Occupational Health, Public Relations, X-ray standards, careers, etc.	Office.	Limited company.	Yes.

Section Two: *Practice*

Conditions treated	Methods	Patient's GP informed of treatment?	Referral by GP	Concurrent treatment	Ethical code
Those with a musculo-skeletal component.	Joint-adjusting procedures. Manipulation. Soft-tissue massage, exercises. Corsets, splints, and supports.	Member therapists actively encouraged to inform GP.	Yes.	Yes. States that it does not interfere with orthodox therapy.	Yes.

Section Three: *Training and qualification*

Entry qualifications	Clinical training	Post-graduate training	Examination	Course duration	Qualification	Course approval	Medical input in training
University matriculation. 3 A's including Chemistry, Biology, or Zoology and 5 GCSE qual.	Final year in college clinic 400 hours min. including 40 new patients (2 hours each), 400 treatments (30 minutes each). Supervisor in training year.	Enrolling in university or polytechnic for Masters, Diploma, or Doctorate. Association holds postgraduate studies in specialist areas.	College exams. Written, oral, and practical with practical and oral final by ECU Board. CNAA validated B.Sc. (Hons.) and postgraduate diploma (PGD) External monitoring by Board of Education.	Year 1, 632 hours. Year 2, 680 hours. Year 3, 660 hours. Year 4, 644 hours. Year 5, 1540 hours.	B.Sc. (Hons) and postgraduate diploma (PGD) validated by CNAA. DC after completing graduate programme.	Association and CNAA.	Pathologists, anatomists, paediatricians, neurologists, and geriatricians.

Section Four: *Research*

Research by organization	Research by another organization	Commissioned research	References in peer-reviewed journal	Own journal
Yes—BCA together with the European Chiropractic Union (ECU) funds a range of research projects.	Yes.	Yes—e.g. Meade et al. (MRC) BMJ 1990; 300: 1,431–7	Yes—e.g. Kane et al., Lancet 1974; 1,333–6	Yes (journal).

TABLE 6.8 **International Association of Crystal Healing Therapists** (n = 40)

Section One: *Organization*

Functions of organization.	Details		Premises	Company status	Register of members
	Number of staff	Council/committee structure			
To provide a high standard of professionalism among crystal healers. To enforce a professional code of conduct among all members. To raise public awareness of crystal healing.	—	Voluntary Committee. Umbrella organization—the Confederation of Healing Organizations.	None.	—	Yes.

Section Two: *Practice*

Conditions treated	Methods	Patient's GP informed of treatment?	Referral by GP	Concurrent treatment	Ethical code
All.	Gentle touch of crystals, oils, gem elixirs meditation, counselling.	Yes—by healers and patients.	Occasionally.	Yes.	Yes.

Section Three: Training and qualification

Entry qualifications	Clinical training	Post-graduate training	Examination	Course duration	Qualification	Course approval	Medical input in training
None.	Supervised teaching of students on each other. Training in running a practice.	Advanced courses and demonstrations.	Written, oral, and practical. Setting up a system of external monitoring.	100 hours contact teaching plus 6 months home study.	Certificate from approved institute. Lay membership by application and fee.	Approved by Association. Trainers must be crystal therapists for 5 years.	None—but course includes basic knowledge of anatomy and physiology.

Section Four: Research

Research by organization	Research by another organization	Commissioned research	References in peer-reviewed journal	Own journal
No.	No.	No.	Yes—*Journal of Alternative and Complementary Medicine*.	Yes (newsletter).

TABLE 6.9 The Aetherius Society

Section One: *Organization*

Functions of organization	Details		Council/committee structure	Premises	Company status	Register of members
	Number of staff					
Spiritual and educational organization engaged in teaching and practice of healing and various metaphysical sciences and aspects of yoga.	3 full-time staff. 40 part-time voluntary staff.		Committee and Board of International Directors.	Headquarters in London and 8 regional centres in the UK.	—	Yes.

Section Two: *Practice*

Conditions treated	Methods	Patient's GP informed of treatment?	Referral by GP	Concurrent treatment	Ethical code
Any conditions.	Spiritual healing through the laying on of hands; absent healing through a yogic form of prayer; colour healing.	No.	Infrequently.	Yes—above therapies do not conflict with medication.	No (ethics taught but not published in the form of a Code of Ethics).

Section Three: *Training and qualification*

Entry qualifications	Clinical training	Post-graduate training	Examination	Course duration	Qualification	Course approval	Medical input in training
None.	None.	Refresher courses—plus opportunity to practice under supervision.	None.	10 hours. Home study of healing textbook required. In-house courses.	None.	None.	None.

Section Four: *Research*

Research by organization	Research by another organization	Commissioned research	References in peer-reviewed journal	Own journal
No.	No.	No.	No.	No.

TABLE 6.10 Confederation of Healing Organizations (n = 8,500)

Section One: *Organization*

Functions of organization	Details		Premises	Company status	Register of members
	Number of staff	Council/committee structure			
Make healing available on the NHS and in private medicine, preferably as a complementary service to orthodox medicine.	One paid part-time secretary. Elected Chairman, Secretary/Treasurer, and consultant.	Council with representative from each of 14 member Associations.	Rented office.	Registered charity.	Compiled for publication in 1993.

Section Two: *Practice*

Conditions treated	Methods	Patient's GP informed of treatment?	Referral by GP	Concurrent treatment	Ethical code
All conditions.	Contact and distant healing.	Patients advised by members to inform GP.	Yes—increasingly so. In 1992 the government clarified its policy on recognition of complementary therapists and the GMC's rules, giving discretionary authority to FHSAs (and GP fund-holders) to pay for Health Promotion Clinics using healers.	In all circumstances—but doctor retains ultimate responsibility for patient management.	Yes.

Section Three: *Training and qualification*

Entry qualifications	Clinical training	Post-graduate training	Examination	Course duration	Qualification	Course approval	Medical input in training
No academic qualifications but character references essential.	None.	None.	Continuous assessment, interviews, and patients' testimonials.	Varies—probationary period of approx. 2 years.	Certificate from individual organization. Working towards acceptances of healing as a NVQ.	Each organization monitors own training with minimum standards set by CHO.	Not mandatory.

Section Four: *Research*

Research by organization	Research by another organization	Commissioned research	References in peer-reviewed journal	Own journal
Various, e.g. cataract trial (no references).	Yes—e.g. ulcers.	Yes—e.g. arthritis.	No.	No—but members associations produce own newsletters.

TABLE 6.11 General Council and Register of Consultant Herbalists (n = 110)

Section One: *Organization*

Functions of organization	Details — Number of staff	Council/committee structure	Premises	Company status	Register of members
Professional association of herbalists and/or homoeopaths in private practice. A training school in herbal therapies and homoeopathy.	Salaried company secretary. 1 part-time clerical assistant. 11 tutorial staff.	Elected Council.	Registered office.	Limited company.	Yes.

Section Two: *Practice*

Conditions treated	Methods	Patient's GP informed of treatment?	Referral by GP	Concurrent treatment	Ethical code
All except diabetes, notifiable diseases, malignant disease, and acute emergencies.	Traditional herbal medicine; homoeopathy, naturopathy; psychotherapy; osteopathy; physiotherapy.	Yes—patients advised to inform GP and herbalists will contact GP.	Yes.	After consulting GP.	Yes.

Section Three: *Training and qualification*

Entry qualifications	Clinical training	Post-graduate training	Examination	Course duration	Qualification	Course approval	Medical input in training
None.	100 hours min. in 2-hour blocks at various clinics.	Annual conference. Newsletter (quarterly).	Written and practical. Council controls—no external validation.	Modular and distant learning.	Registration in association on completing training of Faculty of Herbal Medicine.	Approved and monitored by Council.	None.

Section Four: *Research*

Research by organization	Research by another organization	Commissioned research	References in peer-reviewed journal	Own journal
No.	No.	No.	Yes—too numerous to mention.	No longer.

TABLE 6.12 National Institute of Medical Herbalists (n = 300)

Section One: *Organization*

Functions of organization	Details		Premises	Company status	Register of members
	Number of staff	Council/committee structure			
To regulate and develop the practice of herbal medicine by members. To represent and promote the practice of herbal medicine to the public. To encourage and undertake research.	Two paid part-time administrative staff, managed by the honorary general secretary.	Council—President and 10 Council members elected annually at AGM. Council is voluntary. Sub-structure of Council, e.g. Exam Board, Professional Ethics Committee.	Office.	—	Yes.

Section Two: *Practice*

Conditions treated	Methods	Patient's GP informed of treatment?	Referral by GP	Concurrent treatment	Ethical code
Mainly chronic, some acute. Typically—atopic, digestive, arthritic, gynaecological, and skin conditions; stress, migraines, etc.; and chronic infections.	Consultation on herbal medicine.	Not routinely.	Rarely.	Yes.	Comprehensive

Section Three: *Training and qualification*

Entry qualifications	Clinical training	Post-graduate training	Examination	Course duration	Qualification	Course approval	Medical input in training
Graduates of School of Phytotherapy. GCSE and Chemistry and Biology 'A' Levels (or equivalent).	500 hours. At least 80% of training from clinics at school.	Seminars. Annual conferences. Workshops.	Written, oral, and practical. Clinicals and vivas monitored by external examiners who are medically qualified.	3 days/week over 4 years. 2 days/week home study. Correspondence 2–3 days/week plus summer school of 35 hours.	Graduate of School of Phytotherapy.	Institute monitors final examination. Correspondence course accredited by British Council for Accreditation of Correspondence Courses. Looking at development of course.	Teaching of orthodox medical sciences including differential diagnosis and clinical examination skills. Curriculum development.

Section Four: *Research*

Research by organization	Research by another organization	Commissioned research	References in peer-reviewed journal	Own journal
Yes—linked with the Centre of Complementary Health Studies at the University of Exeter.	Yes—as before.	Yes.	Yes—journals such as *Plant Medicine, Journal of Ethnopharmacology.*	Yes.

Table 6.13 Faculty of Homoeopathy (n = 720)

Section One: Organization

Functions of organization	Details		Premises	Company status	Register of members
	Number of staff	Council/committee structure			
Teaching and practice of homoeopathy to qualified medical practitioners, veterinary surgeons, and dentists.	1 full-time secretary and 5 administrative staff.	Executive and Council.	Premises at the Royal London Homoeopathic Hospital.	Limited company set up under Faculty of Homoeopathy Act 1950.	Yes.

Section Two: Practice

Conditions treated	Methods	Patient's GP informed of treatment?	Referral by GP	Concurrent treatment	Ethical code
All.	Homoeopathic medicine [for definition, see glossary].	Yes—patients advised to inform GPs and by members themselves.	Always.	Allopathic and homoeopathic treatments often taken concurrently.	Yes.

Section Three: *Training and qualification*

Entry qualifications	Clinical training	Post-graduate training	Examination	Course duration	Qualification	Course approval	Medical input in training
Qualified doctors, dentists, and veterinary surgeons.	Yes—at the Royal London Homoeopathic Hospital.	Advanced courses and seminars.	Written, oral and clinical examination.	Range from short introductory courses to a 6-month full-time course.	Member of Faculty of Homoeopathy.	Approved by Council of Faculty of Homoeopathy.	Yes: all teaching is by qualified doctors.

Section Four: *Research*

Research by organization	Research by another organization	Commissioned research	References in peer-reviewed journal	Own journal
Yes—various.	No.	Yes.	Yes—e.g. *BMJ* 1989; 299; 365–6; Lancet 1988; 1,528—9.	Yes—British Homoeopathic Journal.

TABLE 6.14 Society of Homoeopaths (n = 550)

Section One: *Organization*

Functions of organization	Details		Council/committee structure	Premises	Company status	Register of members
	Number of staff					
To develop and maintain high standards for the practice of homoeopathy, including the maintenance of a Register of homoeopaths, and to promote education and training. To promote public awareness of homoeopathy and to encourage its responsible use in the home. To protect the public's freedom to have homoeopathic treatment now and in the future. To regulate and discipline the practice of its practitioner members.	1 full-time general secretary. 1 full-time admin. assistant. 1 full-time office clerk. 1 part-time treasurer. 1 part-time membership secretary.		Board of Directors (usually 9) elected by membership at AGM.	Permanent rented office.	Limited company.	Yes.

Section Two: *Practice*

Conditions treated	Methods	Patient's GP informed of treatment?	Referral by GP	Concurrent treatment	Ethical code
Wide range of acute and chronic, physical, mental, and emotional illness.	Recognized procedures of homoeopathic practice [for definition of homoeopathy, see Glossary].	Yes, with consent of patient.	Small but increasing rate of recommendation by doctor.	In most circumstances.	Yes.

Section Three: *Training and qualification*

Entry qualifications	Clinical training	Post-graduate training	Examination	Course duration	Qualification	Course approval	Medical input in training
Usually a minimum of 5 GCSE and 2 'A' levels.	Students required to complete at least 150 hours of in-clinic supervised practice. Submit full documented evidence of all patients treated and the long-term management of at least six chronic cases.	Seminars run by Society.	A full range of assessment procedures from ongoing course assessments to final written and clinical examinations are used. All colleges employ external examiners in their assessment protocols.	3 years full-time equivalent to undergraduate degree requirements. 4 years part-time min. 120 hours lecture per annum. 15–20 hours week home study.	Regd. membership R.S.Hom is conferred on those licensed graduates who have successfully completed minimum of 1 years supervised practice and examination, clinical course work, management of long-term cases, and a satisfactory site visit to assess the applicant's competence.	Currently being investigated by the Society through the establishment of an Accreditation Board.	All college core curricula contain minimum requirements for instruction in medical sciences. Such teaching is done by qualified medical doctors.

Section Four: *Research*

Research by organization	Research by another organization	Commissioned research	References in peer-reviewed journal	Own journal
Yes—e.g. survey of membership 1991.	Yes—e.g. University of Keele.	No.	Yes—e.g. *Lancet* 1986; 2: 881–6.	Yes.

TABLE 6.15 National Council of Psychotherapists and Hypnotherapy Register (n = 180)

Section One: *Organization*

Functions of organization	Details — Number of staff	Council/committee structure	Premises	Company status	Register of members
To provide a national professional association to represent and protect the interests of independent practitioners of psychological therapies.	No paid officials—voluntary work.	Committee of Management elected at the AGM.	Registered at Secretary's address.	—	Yes.

Section Two: *Practice*

Conditions treated	Methods	Patient's GP informed of treatment?	Referral by GP	Concurrent treatment	Ethical code
Mainly psychological, some physical.	Psychotherapy, psychoanalysis, and hypnotherapy.	Yes—within bounds of confidentiality.	Frequently.	Under advice from GP.	Yes.

Section Three: *Training and qualification*

Entry qualifications	Clinical training	Post-graduate training	Examination	Course duration	Qualification	Course approval	Medical input in training
Training courses deemed suitable by management committee.	Licentiate members must be in supervision for a minimum of 3 years before eligible for full membership.	Frequent workshops and seminars.	'Open examination' and oral board.	—	Three grades: licentiate; full; and fellow.	Approved by Council.	No.

Section Four: *Research*

Research by organization	Research by another organization	Commissioned research	References in peer-reviewed journal	Own journal
Yes. In conjunction with Research Council for Complementary Medicine.	No.	No.	Many.	Yes. (quarterly).

TABLE 6.16 **British Society of Iridologists** (n = 60)

Section One: *Organization*

Functions of organization	Details		Premises	Company status	Register of members
	Number of staff	Council/committee structure			
To teach the principles and practice of iris diagnosis and herbalism. Acting as main ruling body.	2 full-time. 2 part-time. 2 voluntary. (Several part-time teaching staff).	Committee structure (voluntary services).	Leased office.	Limited by guarantee.	Yes.

Section Two: *Practice*

Conditions treated	Methods	Patient's GP informed of treatment?	Referral by GP	Concurrent treatment	Ethical code
'Constitutional'.	Diet. Herbal medicine.	Only at request of patient.	About 15%.	If on drug treatment, only with GP's consent.	Comprehensive.

Section Three: Training and qualification

Entry qualifications	Clinical training	Post-graduate training	Examination	Course duration	Qualification	Course approval	Medical input in training
None.	25 hours in school and outside facilities.	Seminars. Workshops. Annual conference.	Written, oral, and practical. External monitors for examinations (Head of Chiropractic School).	164 hours for course. 520 hours directed home study. Plus major project assignment 120 hours.	Graduate of AESI/H* training course or 5 years full-time practical experience.	Must meet AESI/H* approval. Under negotiation with some polytechnics.	Some teaching. Comprehensive teaching on all aspects of the eye.

Section Four: Research

Research by organization	Research by another organization	Commissioned research	References in peer-reviewed journal	Own journal
Yes—e.g. 'emotional responses from the iris.' 'Intelligence in school children through iris colour'.	Dr Ali Dagbagh, and colour pupil innervation.	No.	No.	Yes.

Note: * Anglo-European School of Iridology/Herbalism.

TABLE 6.17 Association for Systematic Kinesiology (n = 70)

Section One: Organization

Functions of organization	Details Number of staff	Council/committee structure	Premises	Company status	Register of members
To bring systematic kinesiology as a preventive form of health care to the notice of the public. To promote thorough training and standards in kinesiology. To maintain a register of practitioners using systematic kinesiology.	3 part-time voluntary.	Board of Trustees and Council.	Uses the office premises of the Academy of Systematic Kinesiology.	Registered charity.	Yes.

Section Two: Practice

Conditions treated	Methods	Patient's GP informed of treatment?	Referral by GP	Concurrent treatment	Ethical code
Most conditions, which are not pathological'. Does not attempt to diagnose or treat disease but acts as preventive therapy for conditions such as back pain, digestive problems, stress-related disorders.	Muscle testing to access information about the body. Use of light touch or firm pressure on the reflex points of the body, together with diet, to restore balance.	Responsibility of patient to inform GP.	Yes.	Yes.	Yes.

Section Three: *Training and qualification*

Entry qualifications	Clinical training	Post-graduate training	Examination	Course duration	Qualification	Course approval	Medical input in training
Supporting members: none. Professional members: basic and advanced training in applied kinesiology.	At present, supervised clinical practice not compulsory.	Weekend courses and seminars—continuing education a requirement in order to maintain professional status in the Association.	Oral, written, and practical—external monitoring by member of Council (but training without examination possible for those using kinesiology for self and family use only).	200 hours of class teaching. 140 hours min. of directed home study.	None.	None.	Occasional lectures by medical doctors on contra-indicators to kinesiology methods, etc. A medical doctor also acts as adviser to the Academy of Systematic Kinesiology.

Section Four: *Research*

Research by organization	Research by another organization	Commissioned research	References in peer-reviewed journal	Own journal
Empirical and anecdotal.	No.	No.	Annual research papers from the International College of Applied Kinesiology.	Yes.

TABLE 6.18 London College of Massage

Section One: *Organization*

Functions of organization	Details		Council/committee structure	Premises	Company status	Register of members
	Number of staff	Methods				
Training in massage techniques.	Six.		None.	Self-contained premises, with teaching rooms, treatment rooms, student lounge, and office.	—	Yes.

Section Two: *Practice*

Conditions treated	Methods	Patient's GP informed of treatment?	Referral by GP	Concurrent treatment	Ethical code
Mainly back complaints. Also headaches, stiffness, and tension-related complaints.	Therapeutic massage, based on Swedish techniques, oils and aroma-therapy.	Patients sometimes advised to inform GPs, but GPs not informed by therapists themselves.	Not very frequently, but it has been known for stress-related conditions.	Depends—full case history taken when any medication/GP treatment involved.	Yes— Code of British Complementary Medical Association.

Section Three: *Training and qualification*

Entry qualifications	Clinical training	Post-graduate training	Examination	Course duration	Qualification	Course approval	Medical input in training
None.	Supervised clinic once a month.	Specialized courses in sports injuries, listening skills, and remedial massage.	Practical. Advanced course also tested on anatomy and physiology. No external monitoring.	Beginners course—50 hours. Advanced course—72 hours.	Granted by college.	Approved by college.	No.

Section Four: *Research*

Research by organization	Research by another organization	Commissioned research	References in peer-reviewed journal	Own journal
No.	No.	No.	No.	No.

TABLE 6.19 College of Osteopaths Practitioners Association (n = 162)

Section One: *Organization*

Functions of organization	Details — Number of staff	Council/committee structure	Premises	Company status	Register of members
To promote and maintain the highest standards of training, qualification, and treatment in osteopathic practice.	All officers voluntary. 25 teaching faculty plus external examiners paid on part-time contract basis.	Executive Council and Board of Governors: President, Secretary General, and Treasurer plus 5–7 Council members. Various sub-committees including ethical, finance, membership, and political.	Office—also houses the principal teaching clinic.	Registered charity.	Yes.

Section Two: *Practice*

Conditions treated	Methods	Patient's GP informed of treatment?	Referral by GP	Concurrent treatment	Ethical code
Mainly musculo-skeletal. Also others depending on practitioner.	Manipulation. Diet. Exercise. Counselling.	GPs sometimes informed of treatment.	Yes.	Yes.	Yes.

Section Three: *Training and qualification*

Entry qualifications	Clinical training	Post-graduate training	Examination	Course duration	Qualification	Course approval	Medical input in training
Minimum 4 GCSE and 2 'A' Levels in science subjects. (Science foundation course available for those not holding science 'A' Levels).	1,500 hours at least. 600 hours in College clinic.	Mid-year and annual seminars.	Written, oral, and practical plus submission of a thesis.	Weekend teaching and directed home study. Teaching 2,800 hours. Home study 1,000 hours.	Diploma of Osteopathy on passing the examinations and acceptance of thesis.	By College and British Accreditation Council.	Lecturers and examiners in special subjects.

Section Four: *Research*

Research by organization	Research by another organization	Commissioned research	References in peer-reviewed journal	Own journal
Yes—in the form of investigations and thesis of students.	No.	No.	Yes (various osteopathic journals in UK and US).	Yes (newsletter').

TABLE 6.20 General Council and Register of Osteopaths

Section One: *Organization*

Functions of organization	Details		Council/committee structure	Premises	Company status	Register of members
	Number of staff					
Maintaining a level of excellence in training, practice, and conduct of osteopaths. Accrediting courses at osteopathic training establishments. Implementing strict rules of conduct and professional behaviour. Promoting to the public and political bodies the osteopathic profession.	3 salaried executives (Secretary, Assistant Secretary, and Education Adviser). 6 secretarial assistants.		Council of 12 Registered Osteopaths elected at AGM plus up to 8 co-opted members. Full Committee sub-structure including Ethics, Education, European and Parliamentary Liaison, Public Relations, Pay Review. Competence Exercise and External Examiners subcommittees.	Office building occupied under 25-year lease.	Company Limited by Guarantee.	Published annually in January with amendment list in August.

Section Two: *Practice*

Conditions treated	Methods	Patient's GP informed of treatment?	Referral by GP	Concurrent treatment	Ethical code
Those affecting the musculo-skeletal system.	Static and dynamic assessment of biomechanics. Active and passive soft-tissue stretching. Passive movement. Progressive joint mobilization. Manipulation. Ergonomic advice and exercises.	Therapist informs GP, with consent of patient.	Yes.	Yes.	Yes.

Section Three: *Training and qualification*

Entry qualifications	Clinical training	Post-graduate training	Examination	Course duration	Qualification	Course approval	Medical input in training
BCNO*: minimum of 2 science 'A' levels or equivalent, or mature student assessment. BSO:† 5 GCE/GCSE including 2 science 'A' levels or suitable BTEC/OND/ONC/HND/HNC or equivalent. EXO#: 2 science 'A' levels and interview. LCOM**: for qualified physicians only; an entrance examination.	BCNO: 1,100 hours. BSO: 1,350 hours. ESO: 1,539 hours. LCOM: 900 hours within a postgraduate course.	BSO: 2-year part-time course leading to Advanced Diploma in Osteopathy. ESO: 2 or 3 sessions a year. BCNO and LCOM joining with above and other osteopathic organizations to form a Continuing Professional Development Board.	All 4 schools have written, oral, and practical examinations, and use external examiners to assess final clinical competence. External examiners' decisions are final.	BCNO: 4 years full-time (3,744 hours). BSO: 4 years full-time (3,455 hours). ESO: 4 years full-time (4,324 hours). LCOM: 13 months (900 hours)	BCNO: B.Sc. (Hons.). BSO: B.Sc. ESO: Diploma of Osteopathy (DO). LCOM: Member of London College of Osteopathic Medicine (MLCOM). Upon successful completion of above courses, a graduate may apply for membership of the GCRO.	1. Academic validation: BCNO: CNAA (and later the University of Westminster). BSO: Open University. ESO: Council of the College. LCOM: Council of the College. 2. Professional accreditation: All the 4 schools are accredited by the GCRO.	BCNO, BSO, and ESO: lectures and demonstrations in specialist subjects, such as pathology and anatomy. Some clinical tutors at the colleges are medically qualified. LCOM: all teachers are medical practitioners.

Section Four: *Research*

Research by organization	Research by another organization	Commissioned research	References in peer-reviewed journal	Own journal
Yes—currently under-taking a competence exercise.	Yes—examples given. e.g.: BSO: the association of head, neck, and shoulder girdle dysfunction and dysphonia.	No.	Yes—many cited, e.g. *Spine* 1990: 15(5); 364–70.	Yes—*Journal of Osteopathic Education,* which publishes a register of research and research papers.
	ESO: a characterization of patients attending the clinic at the ESO.			
	LCOM: an open controlled assessment of osteopathic manipulation in non-specific low back pain.			
	The 4 schools with courses accredited by the GCRO have formed an Intercollegiate Research Group to further research.			

* BCNO—British College of Naturopathy & Osteopathy
† BSO—British School of Osteopathy
‡ ESO—European School of Osteopathy
***LCOM—London College of Osteopathic Medicine

TABLE 6.21 The Natural Therapeutic and Osteopathic Society and Register (n = 85)

Section One: Organization

Functions of organization	Details				Register of members
	Number of staff	Council/committee structure	Premises	Company status	
Governing body of the London School of Osteopathy.	1 part-time secretary (paid).	General Council. Education Council. Disciplinary Committee.	—	Registered charity.	Yes.

Section Two: Practice

Conditions treated	Methods	Patient's GP informed of treatment?	Referral by GP	Concurrent treatment	Ethical code
All conditions treated related to musculo-skeletal system.	Osteopathy.	Yes—by therapist.	Yes.	Yes.	Yes.

Section Three: *Training and qualification*

Entry qualifications	Clinical training	Post-graduate training	Examination	Course duration	Qualification	Course approval	Medical input in training
London School of Osteopathy (LSO). Degree course 2 science 'A' Levels.	1,401 hours. Outpatient study within the school. Placement with assigned osteopath.	Formal post-graduate courses and *ad hoc* seminars provided by NTOS and LSO.	Written, oral, and practical (plus submission and acceptance of a thesis).	Academic time at weekends. Clinical work over 5 years. Academic 1,170 hours, plus 32 hours field trips. Clinical 1,000 hours. Private study 2,707 hours.	Diploma in osteopathy from approved school.	At present by the Natural Therapeutic and Osteopathic Society (NTOS).	Lecturers and examiners in special subjects and diagnosis. Input of medical studies by specialists in their own field.

Section Four: *Research*

Research by organization	Research by another organization	Commissioned research	References in peer-reviewed journal	Own journal
Yes.	—	No.	No.	Yes. (membership newsletter).

TABLE 6.22 British Biomagnetics Association (n = 100)

Section One: *Organization*

Functions of organization	Details		Council/committee structure	Premises	Company status	Register of members
	Number of staff					
To train osteopaths, acupuncturists, and homoeopaths as well as GPs in the techniques of Biomagnetics.	—		Informal voluntary group.	—	—	Yes.

Section Two: *Practice*

Conditions treated	Methods	Patient's GP informed of treatment?	Referral by GP	Concurrent treatment	Ethical code
Various.	Use of magnets on acupuncture meridians to provide spinal and pelvic alignment.	Not necessarily.	Not known, but many members are GPs.	Most patients are taking prescribed medication.	No.

Section Three: *Training and qualification*

Entry qualifications	Clinical training	Post-graduate training	Examination	Course duration	Qualification	Course approval	Medical input in training
None.	N/A.	Updating courses.	Oral and practical. No external monitoring.	Part-time modular; 45 teaching hours in total.	Granted by Association.	By parent organization—PUPATION OF ITOH AREAS of Japan	Yes—by students.

Section Four: *Research*

Research by organization	Research by another organization	Commissioned research	References in peer-reviewed journal	Own journal
Yes—PIA Japan, parent organization.	No.	No.	No.	Yes.

TABLE 6.23 Confederation of Radionics and Radiesthetic Organizations (n = 120)

Section One: *Organization*

Functions of organization	Details		Council/committee structure	Premises	Company status	Register of members
	Number of staff					
Sharing knowledge. Co-ordinating competences and standards of training. Creating an interface with government/medical profession/public.	—		Secretariat provided by Maperton Trust. Each member organization provides one representative to meet four times a year.	At Maperton Trust.	Registered charity (under Maperton Trust).	Yes.

Section Two: *Practice*

Conditions treated	Methods	Patient's GP informed of treatment?	Referral by GP	Concurrent treatment	Ethical code
All—concerned with the overall health of patient. Takes account of any named disease state.	Uses instrumentation to provide specific corrective energies to the patient through contact, medication, or broadcasting at a distance.	Patients advised to inform own GPs.	Yes.	Yes.	No.

Section Three: *Training and qualification*

Entry qualifications	Clinical training	Post-graduate training	Examination	Course duration	Qualification	Course approval	Medical input in training
'A'-Level Biology or GCSE Human Biology mandatory.	Comparison of training competence being assessed in the 3 member associations.	Seminars. Conferences. Quarterly newsletters.	Written, oral, and practical. No external monitoring.	3–4 years. 800–1,000 hours home study, plus clinical experience, day tutorials, and specialist courses. 2 years as licentiate under supervision.	Membership of Delawarr Society for Radionics.	Course approval by Membership Board. External monitoring under consideration.	Little input. Some lectures and conferences with medical practitioners.

Section Four: *Research*

Research by organization	Research by another organization	Commissioned research	References in peer-reviewed journal	Own journal
Yes—via Delawarr Laboratories Ltd—and the Maperton Trust. Currently limited to basic agriculture research and new instrumentation.	Yes—by manufacturers of instruments.	No.	'Believe so—details not known.'	Yes.

TABLE 6.24 Institute of Signalysis Practitioners (n = 56, inc. 22 medical practitioners)

Section One: *Organization*

Functions of organization	Details				Register of members
	Number of staff	Council/committee structure	Premises	Company status	
'General advancement of the science and art of Signalysis therapy.'	Four?	Administration provided by officers.	Leased office.	Limited company.	Yes.

Section Two: *Practice*

Conditions treated	Methods	Patient's GP informed of treatment?	Referral by GP	Concurrent treatment	Ethical code
'Holistic treatment'—treat patient, not condition.	Signalysis therapy by blood and urine samples—with 'other therapies', such as acupuncture or oxygen therapy.	Yes—with consent of patient.	Frequently.	Yes with agreement of 'other practitioner'.	No.

Section Three: *Training and qualification*

Entry qualifications	Clinical training	Post-graduate training	Examination	Course duration	Qualification	Course approval	Medical input in training
Medical doctors or 'qualified Natural Medicine Practitioners'.	Yes.	3 weekend seminars in each year.	Written, oral, and practical. No external monitoring.	32 hours.	Granted by Institute.	Approved by Institute.	Some.

Section Four: *Research*

Research by organization	Research by another organization	Commissioned research	References in peer-reviewed journal	Own journal
Yes—in progress.	No.	No.	No.	No.

TABLE 6.25 Association of Reflexologists (n = 900)

Section One: *Organization*

Functions of organization	Details				Register of members
	Number of staff	Council/committee structure	Premises	Company status	
To set and maintain standards of reflexology, provide the public with a register of qualified reflexologists, to encourage and accredit training courses, and to give support, further education, a forum, and insurance to members.	Part-time paid administrator, book-keeper, secretary, and co-ordinator.	Council of 12 members consisting of voluntary officers and subcommittees.	—	—	Yes.

Section Two: *Practice*

Conditions treated	Methods	Patient's GP informed of treatment?	Referral by GP	Concurrent treatment	Ethical code
Whole person treated.	Compression techniques using reflexes in hands and feet.	Patients advised to inform own GP.	Yes.	Yes—if any doubt, obtain consent of patient's GP.	Yes.

Section Three: *Training and qualification*

Entry qualifications	Clinical training	Post-graduate training	Examination	Course duration	Qualification	Course approval	Medical input in training
Over 18.	At training establishment.	Quarterly meetings by Association and training establishments.	Oral. Written. Practical.	120+ hours part-time/modular.	Qualified Practitioners of Reflexology.	Assessment Committee and an assessor who visits training establishments.	Anatomy and physiology and occasional medical lecturers.

Section Four: *Research*

Research by organization	Research by another organization	Commissioned research	References in peer-reviewed journal	Own journal
Yes—tinnitus.	No.	No.	Yes.	Yes.

TABLE 6.26 **British Reflexology Association** (n = 420)

Section One: *Organization*

Functions of organization	Details		Premises	Company status	Register of members
	Number of staff	Council/committee structure			
To act as a representative body for people practising reflexology as a profession.	4 administrative (paid honorarium).	Council of 10 members.	Office in conjunction with Bayly School of Reflexology Ltd.	Limited company.	Yes.

Section Two: *Practice*

Conditions treated	Methods	Patient's GP informed of treatment?	Referral by GP	Concurrent treatment	Ethical code
Most—excluding infections and thrombosis.	Reflexology—massage of pressure points in feet.	Patient advised to inform GP.	Occasionally.	Yes, with permission of doctor.	Yes.

Section Three: *Training and qualification*

Entry qualifications	Clinical training	Post-graduate training	Examination	Course duration	Qualification	Course approval	Medical input in training
None but four GCSE advisable.	Unsupervised clinical training 36 hours.	Refresher courses.	Written, practical. No external monitoring.	24 hours lectures. 20 hours practical. 36 hours case studies. Home study.	Certificate to successful students.	Approved by Institute of Complementary Medicine.	36 hours unsupervised clinical training. No indication of medical input.

Section Four: *Research*

Research by organization	Research by another organization	Commissioned research	References in peer-reviewed journal	Own journal
Yes—survey of practitioners plus ongoing review of use of reflexology treatment by nursing staff in QEH, Birmingham.	No.	No.	No.	Yes.

TABLE 6.27 Shiatsu Society (n =165)

Section One: *Organization*

Functions of organization	Details		Council/committee structure	Premises	Company status	Register of members
	Number of staff					
To advance Shiatsu as a healing therapy throughout the UK and elsewhere and to maintain high standards in its practice.	1 full-time administrator.		'Core group' of 5–9 officers elected by membership at AGM.	Office.	—	Yes.

Section Two: *Practice*

Conditions treated	Methods	Patient's GP informed of treatment?	Referral by GP	Concurrent treatment	Ethical code
Range of conditions including migraine, asthma, bronchitis, depression, and circulatory problems.	Bodywork; pressure; tonification and relaxation techniques; healing power; stretching; exercise; using pressure points and energy channels known as 'meridians'; and the Yin-Yang oriental diagnostic system.	Patients advised to inform GP.	Yes—infrequently, but increasing.	Only with consent of patient and in full knowledge of the medication prescribed.	Yes.

Section Three: *Training and qualification*

Entry qualifications	Clinical training	Post-graduate training	Examination	Course duration	Qualification	Course approval	Medical input in training
None.	Minimum of 100 clinical case studies.	Intensive refresher courses.	Oral and practical with letters of nomination.	3 years' study with recognized teachers and total of 500 hours of formal tuition.	3 stages: a) ordinary member; b) registered practitioner (MRSS); c) registered teacher.	Society does not validate courses at schools, but assesses individual teachers by means of the Society's Assessment Panel.	Yes— informal.

Section Four: *Research*

Research by organization	Research by another organization	Commissioned research	References in peer-reviewed journal	Own journal
Informal research undertaken by individuals.	No.	TPA—Consulting Group Ltd.	No.	Yes (newsletter).

7 Good practice in non-conventional therapies

7.1. Discussion of results

In analysing the results from our small survey, it can be seen that the data give rise to more questions than they answer. For instance, several organizations claim to treat 'all conditions' while others have localized and well-defined areas of competence. While direct comparison between organizations is not always helpful, given the very different practices and methods employed, it is salutary to note the elements of best practice which may have wider application to different therapies. These can be divided into the main categories given in the questionnaire: organization (including registration); professional standards; training and qualifications; and research.

7.1.1. Organization

Respondents gave details of very different organizational structures, ranging from a complex infrastructure of democratically elected committees and representatives to small organizations with self-appointed executives. Resources and membership size will dictate to a large extent the scale of organization possible in terms of staff size and premises. Whatever their size, some form of written constitution and forum at which elected members may determine policy is desirable for all representative bodies.

Perhaps the single most important feature of the organization is its registering capacity. The maintenance of a single register of suitably qualified practitioners, which is accessible to the public, provides the greatest safeguard against possible harm to the individual. The present state of affairs, with more than one registering body for many therapies, is not helpful to patients or indeed to members themselves.

One of the distinguishing features of a profession is the existence of a register of members open to public inspection. As stated in the Medical Act of 1858, 'it is expedient that persons requiring medical aid should be enabled to distinguish qualified from unqualified medical practitioners'.[1] The establishment of the General Medical Council in 1858 ensured the maintenance of an official list of practitioners who had achieved agreed minimum standards of medical education. This register was to be regularly updated and open to public scrutiny. Patients could then be protected from unqualified practitioners or those who had been removed from the register for reasons of professional misconduct or gross incompetence.

In terms of non-conventional therapies today, registration of practitioners may take different forms. Those therapies in which the diagnostic process is integral to the application of the therapy, or whose practice involves invasive or potentially harmful techniques, should be subject to a *statutory* register of members. (Official registration of non-conventional therapies will require legislation and resources. These monies should be generated *in addition to* existing levels of funding for health-care services in the UK.) It would probably be sufficient for other therapies to be subject to *voluntary* registration, in which the regulating body for each therapy as a matter of good practice keeps a register of members. In order for public registers of any form—statutory or voluntary—to be meaningful, it is necessary for each therapy to determine the appropriate educational and training needs of members and to set these down as a condition of registration. It is important that such registers be maintained faithfully, as such an instrument has no value without up-to-date and accurate information.

7.1.2. *Professional standards*

Professional standards comprise both the setting of well-defined criteria of clinical competence and the adherence and enforcement of ethical codes of conduct.

Levels of *competence* need to be established for the safe and proficient practice in each therapy. In 1989 the National Council for Vocational Qualifications developed guide-lines with the Training Agency (formerly the Manpower Services Commission)[2] on defining standards of performance or competence. The aim was to produce criteria for standards in a given work setting. The Training Agency established a general protocol for developing competences—or functional analyses—for a given field, consisting of the following stages:

1. determine the limits of the occupational area and the details of the occupations covered;
2. define the key purpose of the occupational area as a whole;
3. find out what relevant materials already exist, including work that people in other sectors might be doing;
4. use groups of expert practitioners to carry out a functional analysis of the area, starting with the key purpose and working from the top down, using a whole role model of competence;
5. identify units and elements from the analysis;
6. check the nation-wide applicability of the units, elements, and their performance criteria, probably by a questionnaire survey;
7. field-test the standards in typical assessment situations to determine whether they can be interpreted with adequate consistency; and
8. provide a mechanism for refining and updating the standards.

Working from this basic model, a competence exercise has been initiated by the General Council and Register of Osteopaths (GCRO); this is still being developed and is therefore subject to change. The detailed report is the product of extensive consultation and piloting with large numbers of osteopathic practitioners. The seven areas identified by the GCRO for competence in osteopathy are in organizing and managing the practice; using palpation; evaluating the patient; planning the treatment of a patient or referring the patient on to another agency; treating the patient; examining progress and re-evaluating the patient; and professional self-management. Full details of the first competence in organizing and managing a practice are given in Appendix 5, as the information may provide a useful model for other therapies. It should be noted that, as with Step 8 identified by the Training Agency above, all standards should be subject to continuous audit and review. Such competences are not permanent fixtures and may need to be revised in the light of changing knowledge and practice.

Practitioners should draw up clear protocols for communicating with medical practitioners and with other therapists. In order to do this, it is essential that therapies should not only establish standards and competences, as detailed above, but also the *limits* of competence. Therapists should be aware of which conditions and individuals they are not able to treat and when patients should be directed to medically qualified practitioners. Patients presenting directly to the therapist without consulting their general practitioner should be encouraged to inform their GP that they are undergoing treatment and, where appropriate, to attend their GP for review at appropriate intervals. It is also essential that non-conventional therapists should not alter the medication or treatment prescribed for patients by their medical practitioner. These issues of communication and responsible management of patients are a necessary part of maintaining professional standards within a therapy and ensuring a constructive dialogue between the different professions responsible for patient care.

Each therapy should set up an effective and enforceable disciplinary mechanism and a binding code of ethics. These are the two aspects of professional conduct which are necessary to maintain patient confidence and standards of care. It is important not only that the machinery to maintain discipline and professional standards be in place, but also that it is *seen* by individual therapists and members of the public to be effective and applied. To return again to the analogy with the medical profession in the middle of the last century, the 1858 Medical Act provided that practitioners convicted of felony or misdemeanour should have their names erased from the Register, as would any practitioner who 'shall, after due inquiry, be judged by the General Council to have been guilty of infamous conduct in any professional respect'.

Allegations of professional misconduct and malpractice should be thoroughly investigated by an appropriately constituted committee or council and backed up by a suitable range of penalties, with deregistration as the ultimate sanction. In order to be effective, it is essential that the disciplinary mechanism is directly linked to the register, providing safeguards against the continued practising of incompetent practitioners or those in breach of established guide-lines of professional conduct. Mechanisms for patient complaints should be clear and accessible. The Consumers Association has mapped out a model complaints system[3] integrating the key features of visibility, accessibility, flexibility, impartiality, and effectiveness.

Principles of ethical practice should be developed. A code of ethics for practitioners should include guidance on confidentiality; personal relationships between therapists and patients; and relationships with colleagues and other health-care staff. Importantly, claims to 'cure' individuals should be outlawed. The codes of ethics which have accompanied responses to the BMA survey range from a few prescriptive 'rules' of behaviour to more comprehensive guidance on a wide range of aspects of professional conduct.

7.1.3. *Training and qualification*

Examination of the BMA survey response summaries indicate that there is a considerable range of standards, aspirations, and levels of training for practitioners of non-conventional therapies. At one end of the spectrum, discrete clinical disciplines (as defined in Chapter 5) require levels of training commensurate with the responsibilities such therapists have to patients in their care. Training for such disciplines are likely to be degree equivalents. However, there are certain broad principles which could be applied—albeit at different levels for different therapies—to all training programmes for persons who are applying or prescribing forms of non-conventional medicine to patients.

As a primary step, it is essential that each therapy should establish a *core curriculum*, setting out the basic competences required for the practice of that therapy. Courses should be of credible duration and type to provide a practitioner competent in that therapy. Good practice would also suggest that a minimum, core 'basic science/medical' curriculum should be compulsory for all practices claiming to have a therapeutic influence. It should be noted that a foundation anatomy or physiology component is required for the most basic of first-aid courses, and this should be replicated in any practice which has therapeutic claims. This foundation medical/science course might include some very basic knowledge of pharmacology and an appreciation of the hazards in removing patients from prescribed medication, for instance, interrupting a course of antibiotics. Most fundamentally, such a basic course would instil in all practitioners understanding of the ways in which apparently innocent symptoms—often the common ones—can often be indicative of serious disease. This element of core 'medical' knowledge is associated with the need for therapists to establish the limits of their competence, as discussed in Chapter 4, and to be aware of when it is necessary to encourage actively the involvement of the patient's doctor.

Secondly, a regulatory body for a given therapy should assume responsibility for the clinical and professional *accreditation* of training establishments. Developments such as the establishment of the British Acupuncture Accreditation Board (BAAB), to accredit colleges by assessing compliance with established minimum standards in acupuncture, are most encouraging. The BAAB has set out a schedule for the accreditation process, which includes a period in which colleges review their structure and operation with the support of the Board, before being approved as an accredited college. The accreditation status would be renewable, probably every five years.

For a given therapy it should be possible to reach agreement on minimum requirements of training competence. However, these could be achieved while allowing for a certain degree of flexibility. Within agreed parameters, a certain amount of diversity in training establishments is healthy in catering for the individual tastes of students and the different approaches and expertise among the teaching staff.

A rigorous assessment programme should ensure that each training establishment is externally monitored against known assessment criteria. For the discrete clinical disciplines, a level of training commensurate with their responsibilities for patient care is necessary, and it might be expected that graduating students should be able to demonstrate the following levels of competence:

- A sound knowledge of anatomy, physiology, pathology, basic medical therapeutics, and the principles of their own therapeutic modality. The practitioner must also have acquired a sufficient depth of knowledge of the principles of medicine and the pathological process of disease, and be aware of the physiological basis for their treatment and modality.

- The ability to collect relevant information from the taking of an appropriate case history and an examination of the patient enabling the practitioner to formulate an appropriate diagnosis and effective treatment plan, as well as the likely prognosis and any suitable prophylaxis.

- An ability to conduct and interpret a relevant clinical examination and use currently accepted clinical testing procedures as well as an ability to interpret any ancillary tests.

- In reaching a diagnosis, a practitioner must be able to show that he or she has thought differentially using a rationale based upon current knowledge of anatomy, physiology, and pathology, demonstrating that he or she has considered not only the potential contra-indications of treatment but also has an awareness that symptoms manifested by the patient may be emanating from a site or cause distant from the presenting problem, and may be indicative of serious underlying disease.

- The practitioner should demonstrate an awareness of the relevance of a patient's personal life history, including psychological aspects, inherited predispositions, previous medical history, life-style factors, and social and occupational background. This is particularly important so that the patient's own expectations will be considered in formulating a treatment plan.

- Practitioners should show an awareness of limits of competence and the scope of their particular therapy, together with a knowledge of absolute and relative contra-indications to therapy. With this goes the ability to recognize conditions where a particular treatment is inappropriate, and also when a patient is suffering from a condition that requires immediate referral to the patient's GP.

- They should show an awareness of the need to plan a particular course of treatment and be able to anticipate its effectiveness with the patient concerned. A practitioner should be able to communicate his or her findings, diagnosis, prognosis—and prophylaxis, where appropriate—not only to the patient's GP but also to the patient, in such a way that the patient's own expectations are taken into consideration.

- Practitioners should show an awareness of the need to evaluate and monitor the patient's progress in line with the proposed treatment plan and an awareness that, if anticipated outcomes are not met, consideration should be given to referral to the appropriate agency.

A training strategy should also include an appropriate structured, supervised, and monitored clinical training. It is essential that the ethos of 'professional practice' and the basic competences are absorbed during the clinical training at undergraduate level. Such professional training required to equip the practitioner for future practice can be achieved only by extensive and continuous exposure to clinical practice supervised by experienced and suitably trained clinical teaching staff. It is through directed clinical experience that the novice practitioner will acquire full competence and confidence.

A body with responsibility for training should also ensure that programmes of refresher courses and continuing education are available for the practising therapist. This will enable not only familiarity with new techniques and developments, but will also ensure maintenance of standards in existing techniques and practice.

The student of non-conventional therapy must be trained to be a competent practitioner and also be given the basic skills to carry out audit and research, particularly in the discrete clinical disciplines. It is important that students should acquire the basic principles of research methodology at an undergraduate level, so that a research culture is inculcated at an early stage.

7.1.4. Research

The results of the BMA survey indicate that there is an awareness among different non-conventional therapies of the importance of research in establishing a given practice. Although most of the responding organizations answered affirmatively to one or more of the questions dealing with research, very few of the group had either carried out their own research to a standard that resulted in publication in an independent—that is, not an in-house—journal, or had commissioned others to carry out research of this kind. The most convincing evaluations have been carried out for manipulative techniques, particularly for low back and neck pain.

Manipulative techniques

A good example of a large randomized trial is the study by the Medical Research Council comparing chiropractic and orthodox treatment of low back pain. The investigation by Meade and colleagues[4] was presented as a 'pragmatic' randomized controlled trial, in which 741 patients aged between 18 and 65 years were allocated randomly to chiropractic or 'conventional' hospital out-patient treatment. The original study and ensuing correspondence in the *British Medical Journal* raised a number of interesting questions about the methodology for comparison of different treatments. For instance, in administering different forms of manipulative technique, the concept of a double blind trial cannot seriously apply. The willingness of those practising chiropractic methods to submit these techniques to open scrutiny is commendable and it is hoped that this pioneering major study will pave the way for similar research ventures into other non-conventional therapies.

Homoeopathy

Other techniques which have received some evaluation are homoeopathy and acupuncture. Further and very carefully conducted trials of homoeopathy would be particularly helpful.

Although the scientific basis for homoeopathy appears uncertain, further investigation is needed to help resolve the confusion caused by previous trials. The controversy surrounding the assertions made by a group led by the scientist Benveniste in *Nature*[5] and widely reported in the general press has helped to confuse the public about homoeopathic claims. The debate centred on an assertion that 'it is possible to dilute an aqueous solution of an antibody virtually indefinitely without the solution losing its biological activity'.[6] Attempts to account for this observation, which 'strike at the roots of two centuries of observation and rationalization of physical phenomena', provoked further controversy. Subsequent investigations by an independent team suggested that these results were not reproducible and that the original study included systematic errors, including observer bias and poor statistical controls.[7] The fierce controversy aroused by this particular piece of research indicates the need for scrupulous and defensible research into homoeopathy as a basis for further claims.

The recent review by Kleijnen and colleagues of clinical trials in homoeopathy provides a useful basis for further work.[8] Having assessed 107 controlled trials world-wide, the authors concluded that: 'at the moment the evidence from clinical trials is positive but not sufficient to draw definitive conclusions because most trials are of low methodological quality and because of the unknown role of publication bias.' On the basis of these findings, they recommended further investigations into homoeopathy, using 'a few well performed controlled trials in humans with large numbers of participants under rigorous double blind conditions'.

Acupuncture

A number of research studies have been undertaken in the UK and Europe evaluating the use of therapeutic acupuncture.[9] However, the largest body of research into the effects of classical acupuncture exists in the People's Republic of China. These studies have focused on validating the existence of acupuncture channels and points, examining physiological responses to the stimulation of acupuncture points, and carrying out hospital-based clinical research. It is encouraging to note that the Council for Acupuncture has established a research committee to review current literature and work with leaders in the field of acupuncture research and conventional medicine research to construct suitable research designs. Further trials of acupuncture would also be helpful, as recent evidence suggesting that release of endogenous opiates may contribute to the relief of pain and this provides a solid basis for further investigation.[10]

Herbalism

At present, it appears that there have been few controlled trials evaluating the benefits of therapeutic herbal interventions. There have, however, been some reported case histories in medical journals documenting the potential hazards associated with different preparations. A recent report in the *Annals of Internal Medicine*[11] noted the development of hepatitis in patients using the weight-loss herb germander. A similar example was cited in the *Lancet*, where a herbal preparation marketed as a slimming aid was found to contain significant amounts of sparteine, obtained from the broom plant.[12] Excessive doses of sparteine are associated with a number of adverse reactions, including circulatory collapse, respiratory arrest, cramps, and diarrhoea. Anecdotal evidence from the National Poisons Unit of cases noted to date from the recently established reporting system (see Chapter 4) include incidents of lead poisoning in children having used surma, an Indian eye remedy with a lead content of up to 86 per cent. (It should be noted that it has been public health policy for many years to discourage actively the use of surma in this country.) The valuable data collated at the National Poisons Unit will provide much-needed evidence on the adverse effects of different 'natural' preparations, which at present are poorly documented.

Other therapies

With the exception of osteopathy,[13] chiropractic, acupuncture, and homoeopathy, the public and professions should be aware of the paucity of research on the effectiveness and safety of different therapies. Examples of 'pioneer' collaborative research in areas where few studies have been undertaken to date, such as the current study under the auspices of the Royal College of Nursing on nursing and aromatherapy in intensive therapy units, should be encouraged and developed. Some approaches lie at the boundary between conventional and non-conventional medicine. For example, in one study 'biofeedback' techniques appeared to have an effect in lowering blood-pressure in a controlled trial of 200 people with two or more coronary risk factors.[14] While the authors could not dismiss the question of systematic bias in the study, they suggest that relaxation techniques and stress-management training may play a part in the reduction of mild hypertension. Biofeedback methods, together with other relaxation-based behaviourial methods, including yoga, deserve further evaluation.

7.2. Summary

At present there are very few data concerning the practice and control of non-conventional therapies. The British Medical Association undertook a small survey to give representative bodies the opportunity of presenting detailed information on the organization, practice, training, qualifications, and research for various therapies. Detailed analysis of the summaries of survey responses are left to the reader.

The diversity of different practices and organizations is evident from examination of the BMA survey results. However, for all therapies, good practice would demand that each body representing a therapy demonstrate: an organized structure; a single register of members; guide-lines on relationships with medical practitioners; sound training at accredited institutions; an effective ethical code; agreed levels of competence; and a proven commitment to research. Such features not only safeguard the patient from possible harm, but also provide practitioners of the therapy with a recognized status.

8 *Summary and recommendations*

[*Numbers in square brackets after the recommendations refer to fuller discussion of the issue in the main body of the text*]

The term 'non-conventional therapies' covers a wide and diverse range of practices. Some treat particular parts of the body or conditions and others aim to provide complete treatment or therapy for the generality of diseases and patients. It is apparent that different therapies have little in common in the way of aspirations, practice, and tradition. The means of control over these therapies varies widely from country to country within Europe. The Commission of the European Communities has stated emphatically that legislation at EC level is unlikely in coming years in the area of non-conventional therapies. With the possible exception of medicinal products, a uniform system of regulation across Europe is only a remote possibility. The most important influence on the regulation of non-conventional therapies will continue to be national law; the bulk of this report is therefore concerned with developments in the UK.

While no attempt has been made to evaluate different therapies in this report, it is clear that the key to enhancing the credibility of different practices, whether in orthodox medicine or non-conventional therapies, is research. Good-quality research is essential in order to maximize the benefits and minimize the harms of different treatments. There is at present a paucity of systematically collected data on the use and recorded adverse effects of non-conventional therapies. There are areas of orthodox medicine where such information is similarly unavailable. Such evidence, obtained by carefully designed research investigations, is necessary in order to make informed decisions on the risks and benefits of different treatments.

Much of this report is focused on those practices which we have labelled as *discrete clinical disciplines*. These are the therapies which have established foundations of training and have the potential for greatest use alongside orthodox medical care. Our category of discrete clinical disciplines covers the practices of acupuncture, chiropractic, herbalism, homoeopathy, and osteopathy which appear to be the five most common therapies in use in the UK today.

Given the wide diversity in non-conventional therapies, from discrete clinical disciplines through to healing and self-help therapies such as yoga, it is not possible to set out a single model for regulation which would be appropriate for all practices. However, it is hoped that this report will make a positive contribution by highlighting areas of good practice in disciplines which may be emerging or lacking the support of more established therapies. The development of more rigorous means of control and regulation for different therapies can only benefit the patient, which must be the goal for doctors and therapists alike.

8.1. Good practice

It is difficult at present for individuals to be certain that the therapist whom they are consulting is competent to practise. Similarly, it is not easy for doctors to ensure that the therapists to whom they transfer care of patients are competent. The present situation, in which anybody is free to practise, irrespective of their training or experience, is unacceptable. Where individuals undergo courses of training designed to equip them for the practice of particular therapies, these should conform to minimum standards appropriate to the responsibilities and demands of that therapy.

The BMA recommends that a *single* regulating body be established for each therapy. Such organizations should follow best practice in adopting all of the following features:

8.1.1. *Registration*

• A single register of members, open to public scrutiny, entry to which is limited to competent practitioners [7.1.1].

8.1.2. *Professional standards*

- A defined protocol for communicating with medical practitioners and other therapists both within and without their own discipline and a system for maintaining case records of patients/clients [7.1.2];

- clearly understood areas of competence, including limits of competence and contra-indications to treatment [4.4; 7.1.2];

- enforceable ethical code governing all aspects of professional conduct, linked to effective disciplinary mechanism [7.1.2];

- well-publicized and accessible complaints procedure [7.1.2].

8.1.3. *Training*

- Training structure appropriate to the task and of a credible duration at accredited and externally monitored educational establishments [7.1.3];

- all practices claiming to have a therapeutic influence should include in their training courses a foundation in the basic medical sciences [7.1.3];

- consideration should be given to a core curriculum for the training schedule of each therapy including appropriate clinical and medical input [7.1.3];

- limits of competence must be established for each therapy during the training process. Patients suffering from conditions not amenable to treatment must be identified and referred to the appropriate agency. This is particularly important in cases where medical attention is needed [7.1.3];

- provision should be made for continuing education for qualified members, and for refresher courses [7.1.3];

- training in clinical audit, so that practice and management of patients are evaluated rigorously at regular intervals [7.1.3];

8.1.4. *Research*

- Encouragement of professional development and research [7.1.4].

8.2.   Regulation

The criteria above represent best practice which should be the aim of all therapies. However, in order to protect patients, some therapies should be regulated by statute. Those therapies in which the diagnostic process is integral to the application of the therapy, and whose practice involves invasive or potentially harmful techniques, should be subject to regulation by law. The BMA therefore recommends that:

● the case for the statutory self-regulation of each discrete clinical discipline should be considered by an appropriate independent body and, where applicable, appropriate legislation introduced [5.3].

8.3.   Doctors and therapists

Increasing numbers of doctors wish to make use of non-conventional therapies for their patients. A distinction has been made between the powers of referral and of delegation. The doctor refers a patient to another individual to use his or her professional judgement to assess the patient and decide if (and what) treatment is necessary and, where appropriate, to provide that treatment. In the referral model, the general practitioner refers care of the patient to a specialist for the duration of a particular episode of treatment, but will retain clinical responsibility for the overall care of the patient. In delegating care, by contrast, tasks which are routinely performed by the doctor are transferred to another health-care professional, such as a nurse. The doctor remains clinically accountable for the patient during that treatment.

The question arises as to how appropriate the model of delegation is for non-conventional therapies, in particular the discrete clinical disciplines, when the treatment may be outside the scope of the doctor's skill and experience. It may be difficult at present for the doctor to be confident that the practitioner is competent in this area. In the case of therapies which are subject to statutory regulation, such as osteopathy, the onus for determining the clinical competence of the therapist is to a large extent removed from the doctor. The BMA therefore recommends that:

- the General Medical Council be asked to consider whether doctors should be permitted to *refer* patients for specific treatments to registered practitioners in those therapies which are subject to statutory self-regulation [4.1].

8.4. Doctor–therapist communication

Responsibility for complete medical diagnosis and overall management of the patient rests with the patient's general medical practitioner. Paragraph 92 of the current General Medical Council guide-lines states that 'it is in the best interests of patients for one doctor to be fully informed about and responsible for the comprehensive management of a patient's medical care'. The situation where a patient is given advice by a therapist which conflicts with the drug regimen or treatment given by their registered medical practitioner is detrimental to the best interests of the patient. It is essential that proper channels of communication be established between non-conventional therapists and doctors to prevent the occurrence of such a situation. In addition, the doctor should be fully informed of any non-conventional treatment which the patient is receiving. The BMA therefore recommends that:

- therapists should not alter the instructions or prescriptions given by a patient's medical practitioner without prior consultation and agreement with that doctor [4.4];
- doctors should ask about their patients' use of non-conventional therapies whenever they obtain a medical history [4.5].

8.5. Research

Research is extremely valuable in advancing knowledge in a given discipline and in evaluating the benefits and harms of different practices. Research in non-conventional therapies has to date been of inconsistent quality. It is recognized that this is due in part to difficulties in attracting appropriate resources to fund good-quality research. In addition to problems in funding research studies, there have been more general difficulties in inculcating a culture that recognizes research as an essential activity. Recent research initiatives in various non-conventional therapies, such as the national randomized trial of chiropractic, are welcome as an important step in ensuring public and professional confidence in particular modalities. The BMA recommends that:

- Priority should be given to research into acupuncture, chiropractic, herbalism, homoeopathy, and osteopathy as the therapies most commonly used in this country [7.1.4];

- in the absence of research foundations for specific therapeutic disciplines, support be given to organizations such as the Research Council for Complementary Medicine (RCCM) to raise awareness of the need for more research in non-conventional therapies [4.6];

- core curricula for undergraduate training establishments should include components on research methodology, information technology, and statistics [4.6];

- experienced practitioners in different therapies should be encouraged to undertake practice surveys measuring work-load and patient characteristics. Such research could be facilitated by postgraduate training and on-call advice on research protocols from organizations such as the RCCM [4.6].

8.6. Monitoring and surveillance

In order to minimize the potential harms of treatments and maximize the benefits of different treatments, it is important to record any adverse reactions occurring after an intervention. Surveillance schemes are necessary to collate information on incidents which may be used to test the safety and quality of different preparations. The BMA therefore recommends that:

- Continued funding from the Department of Health and the Ministry of Agriculture, Fisheries, and Food be made available for the investigation into adverse reactions to herbal medicines and other preparations at the National Poisons Unit [4.6];

- the Council of Europe Co-operation in Science and Technology (COST) project on non-conventional therapies be approved by the UK government [2.4].

8.7. Medical understanding of non-conventional therapies

Recent surveys suggest that doctors increasingly require more information on non-conventional therapies. Doctors need to know more about different therapies in order to delegate care appropriately, and to advise patients as to the likely benefits and hazards of treatments. Some doctors may even wish to undertake more detailed training in order to practise as a therapist. The BMA in particular recommends that:

- accredited postgraduate sessions be set up to inform clinicians on the techniques used by different therapists and the possible benefits for patients [4.5];

- consideration should be given to the inclusion of a familiarization course on non-conventional therapies within the medical undergraduate curriculum [4.5].

8.8. Medically qualified therapists

It is recognized that particular skills need to be acquired in order to achieve competence in different therapies. The General Medical Council has stated that a question of serious professional misconduct may arise by 'a doctor persisting in unsupervised practice of a branch of medicine without having the appropriate knowledge and skill or having acquired the experience which is necessary'. The BMA therefore recommends that:

- medically qualified practitioners wishing to practise any form of non-conventional therapy should undertake recognized training in that field approved by the appropriate regulatory body, and should only practise the therapy after registration [4.2].

Appendix 1
Contra-indications for osteopathic practice

The osteopath must be aware of his/her limits of competence and be able to recognize when the patient is suffering from a condition where osteopathic treatment may be inappropriate and which accordingly requires referral to a registered medical practitioner. Through clinical reasoning the osteopath will select techniques appropriate to the patient and avoid the use of direct techniques contra-indicated at specific sites.

The following conditions have been identified by the General Council and Register of Osteopaths as those traditionally considered to be contra-indications to direct techniques at the site:

- Primary bone tumours
- Sarcomas
- Metastases
- Fractures
- Recent major trauma without X-ray
- Local infectious conditions (e.g. osteomyelitis)
- Acute inflammatory conditions (e.g. acute osteoarthritis, rheumatoid arthritis, ankylosing spondylitis)
- Aneurysms
- Severe osteophytosis
- Any condition that will introduce ligamentous instability
- Increased pain or radicular symptoms on positioning
- Angiomas
- Active growth disorders
- Pregnancy in the eighth to twelfth weeks
- Haemophilia
- Thrombocytopaenia
- Active phase of MS, ME, AIDS
- Prodromal symptoms (e.g. migraine, epilepsy, viral infections)

- Gross morphological congenital abnormalities (e.g. cervical ribs)
- Metabolic conditions (e.g. osteoporosis, Paget's, Cushing's)
- Prolapsed invertebral disc
- Arterial insufficiency

The above list is an appendix to a section describing the clinical reasoning used by an osteopath to decide contra-indications to treatment.

Source: General Council and Register of Osteopaths, *Competences Required for Osteopathic Practice* (GCRO, Reading, 1992).

Appendix 2
Regional advisers in general practice

North-Western Region
Department of Postgraduate
  Medical Studies
Gateway House
Piccadilly South
MANCHESTER M60 7LP

Northern Region (Scotland)
Postgraduate Medical Centre
Raigmore Hospital
INVERNESS IV2 3UJ

Eastern Region (Scotland)
Postgraduate Division; Level 8
Ninewells Hospital and Medical
  School
DUNDEE DD1 9SY

Army
Department of General Practice
Royal Army Medical College
Millbank
LONDON SW1P 4RJ

Royal Navy
Adviser in General Practice
Royal Naval Sick Quarters
HMS Drake
Devonport
PLYMOUTH
Devon PL2 2BG

Sheffield
Department of Postgraduate
  Medicine
Faculty of Medicine and Dentistry
University of Sheffield Medical
  School
Beech Hill
SHEFFIELD S10 2RX

Northern Ireland Region
Northern Ireland Council for Postgraduate Medical Education
5 Annadale Avenue
BELFAST BT7 3JH

Welsh Region
Postgraduate Department
Riversdale House
Bridgend
MID GLAMORGAN CF31 3NL

North-Eastern Region (Scotland)
Forresterhill Health Centre
Westburn Road
ABERDEEN AB9 2AY

Western Region (Scotland)
West of Scotland Committee for
  Postgraduate Medical Education
The University
GLASGOW G12 8QQ

Royal Air Force
Royal Air Force Dept. of Primary
   Care
Institute of Community and
   Occupational Medicine
RAF Halton
AYLESBURY
Bucks HP22 5PG

South-West Thames Region
British Postgraduate Medical
   Federation
University of Surrey
Stag Hill
GUILDFORD
Surrey GU2 5XH

Liverpool
Postgraduate General Practice
   Office
2nd Floor
Duncan Building
The University PO Box 147
LIVERPOOL L69 3BX

South-Eastern Region (Scotland)
Pfizer Foundation
Hill Square
EDINBURGH EH8 9DR

Northern Region
Division for General Practice
Regional Postgraduate Institute for
   Medicine and Dentistry
The University 11 Framlington
   Place
NEWCASTLE UPON TYNE NE2
   4AB

Yorkshire Region
Postgraduate Dean's Office
First Floor, West Wing
Yorkshire Health Buildings
Park Parade
HARROGATE HG1 5AH

Wessex Region
South Academic Block
Southampton General Hospital
Tremona Road
SOUTHAMPTON SO9 4XY

Oxford Region
The Medical School Offices
John Radcliffe Hospital
Headington
OXFORD OX3 9DU

East Anglia Region
East Anglian Regional Health
   Authority
Union Lane
Chesterton
CAMBRIDGE CB4 1RF

North-West Thames Region
RA in General Practice
Royal Postgraduate Medical School
Commonwealth Building
Hammersmith Hospital
LONDON W12 0HS

North-East Thames Region
British Postgraduate Medical
   Federation
Room 49, West Wing, Nurses' Home
North Middlesex Hospital
LONDON N18 1QX

South-East Thames Region
Regional Adviser in General
   Practice
Department of General Practice
Guy's Hospital Medical School
St Thomas Street
LONDON SE1 9RT

Leicester
Postgraduate Office
University of Leicester
School of Medicine
Glenfield General Hospital
LEICESTER LE3 9QP

Nottingham
Postgraduate Office
Medical School
Queen's Medical Centre
NOTTINGHAM NG7 2UH

South-Western Region
The University
Medical Postgraduate Department
Canynge Hall
Whiteladies Road
BRISTOL BS8 2PR

March 1993

Devon/Cornwall
Department of General Practice
Exeter Postgraduate Medical School
Barrack Road
EXETER EX2 5DW

West Midlands Region
West Midlands Regional Health
   Authority
1 Vernon Road
Edgbaston
BIRMINGHAM B16 9SA

Appendix 3
Further reading in research methods

Individual practitioners wishing to undertake research in aspects of non-conventional therapies should be encouraged to do so by their regulating body. Medical practitioners should seek funding and support from their local Regional Health Authority Research and Development Committees. All individuals carrying out investigations into aspects of health care should be properly trained in research methodology, statistics, survey or experiment design, and data analysis. As a starting-point, it may be helpful to make use of the following titles, which were written in the main part for medical practitioners undertaking research:

D. Armstrong, M. Calnan, and J. Grace, *Research Methods for General Practitioners* (Oxford University Press, Oxford, 1990).

J. G. R. Howie, *Research in General Practice*, 2nd edn. (Chapman & Hall, London, 1989).

M. J. Gardner and D. G. Altman, *Statistics with Confidence* (British Medical Journal Publishing, London, 1989).

G. Rose and D. J. P. Barker, *Epidemiology for the Uninitiated*, 2nd edn. (British Medical Journal Publishing, London, 1986).

T. D. V. Swinscow, *Statistics at Square One*, 7th edn. (British Medical Journal Publishing, London, 1982).

S. J. W., 'Good surveys guide', *BMJ*, 302 (1991), 302–3.

Appendix 4
BMA questionnaire schedule

Survey of non-conventional therapies

Please give answers as simply and briefly as possible. Additional material (for example, course curricula) and any general comments should be attached separately.

1 Organization

a) Name:

b) Main address:

c) Contact person:

d) Number of practising members:

e) What are the functions of your organization?

f) Please give details of how your organization operates (append answer on separate sheet)

    e.g. Is there a Council or committee structure?

           Details of staff, if any (indicating numbers full-time/part-time and whether paid or voluntary):

           Details of premises from which organization operates:

g) Does your organization maintain a register of recognized practitioners?

yes/no

2 Practice

Please outline the methods and variety of treatments used by practitioners registered with your organization.

a) What conditions or complaints do your practitioners treat?

b) What method(s) do your practitioners mainly use?

c) Are those patients treated by your members advised to inform their GP that they are undergoing therapy?

Do your members themselves inform GPs of patients they have treated?

d)   Please indicate if patients are ever referred to your practitioners by general practitioners. If so, how frequently?

e)   In what circumstances can your practitioners treat patients who are concurrently taking a course of prescribed medication?

f)   Do you have a code of ethics for your members?   yes/no
     If YES, please enclose a copy and explain your disciplinary procedures.

3   Training

Please give details of training institutions associated with your organization and any other courses which qualify practitioners for membership of your organization.

a)   What are the educational aims and objectives of such course(s) and what standards of competence are required of graduates?

b)   What are the procedures for validation and accreditation of these courses by your organization? What other means are there of external validation for these course(s)?

c)   How does your organization monitor standards of training at these establishments?

d)   How is the course structured, e.g. full-time/part-time/modular?

e)   Please give indication of the total number of teaching contact hours, both academic and clinical.
     In addition, please provide information on any *directed* home study.

f)   For clinical training, indicate how many hours of supervised clinical training (with patients) is necessary; does this take place in a clinic attached to the school or other facilities?

g)   Is there any input into the course by registered medical practitioners?
                                                                        yes/no
     If YES, what form does this input take?

h)   Are there facilities for continuing education and/or updating?   yes/no
     If YES, what form do these take?

4   Qualifications

a)   What are the minimum requirements for membership of your organization?

b)   Are these qualifications conferred after examination?   yes/no
     If YES, what form does the final examination take? Written/Oral/Practical

c)   Is there a process of external monitoring for these final exams? If YES, by whom?

d)   Are these qualifications conferred by:
    your organization   yes/no
    another organization (e.g. CNAA)   yes/no
    If YES, please specify which organization.

5   Research

a)   Is your organization carrying out any research itself or has it done so in the past?   yes/no
If YES, please give brief details and references.

b)   Is another organization or associated school carrying out research on your techniques or have done in the past?   yes/no
If YES, please give brief details and references.

c)   Has any organization been commissioned to carry out research on your behalf?   yes/no
If YES, please give brief details and references.

d)   Has your therapy been evaluated in studies leading to publications in peer-reviewed (refereed) journals?   yes/no
If YES, please give references (*excluding* reviews, editorials, and letters that do not include original data).

e)   Does your organization or related organizations produce a journal or other publication?   yes/no
If YES, please enclose a sample.

THANK YOU FOR YOUR HELP

Appendix 5
Organizing and managing the practice

Source: General Council and Register of Osteopaths, *Competences Required for Osteopathic Practice* (1992).

Different specifications will clearly need to be drawn up for the various therapies. However, there are certain common threads in defining a competent practitioner for all types of therapy. These broad areas of competence will include such components as the organization and management of a practice; the evaluation of patients (including taking of case histories and making appropriate referrals to other health-care staff); treatment of patients; and examining and re-evaluating the progress of the patient.

Outlined below is a detailed check-list of just one aspect of competence, the running of a practice. This represents best practice which should be adopted by most practising therapists. It is recognized that some of these requirements may not be practicable for those working in smaller practices; however, these considerations should be borne in mind.

Competence to organize and manage the practice

To demonstrate acceptable standards of competence, the therapist will have to be able to:

a) Identify and define the needs and requirements for a fully operational practice.
   And in particular to:
   i. Select an appropriate location and site, considering accessibility.
   ii. Estimate costs.
   iii. Formulate a budget to include borrowing, insurance, pensions.
   iv. Select premises with a suitable treatment room and associated facilities including WC and changing area.
   v. Select the furnishing and equipment and consider decor.

    vi.   Identify staffing needs.

    vii.   Anticipate what liaison is needed with other health professionals.

    viii.   Provide appropriate means for reception of patients.

b) Maintain financial records in compliance with legal requirements.
And in particular to:

    i.   Use double-entry bookkeeping.

    ii.   Indicate fees collected/outstanding.

    iii.   Record outgoings.

    iv.   Record taxation disbursements (NI, VAT, Income Tax).

    v.   Record insurance payments.

    vi.   Record pension payments.

    vii.   Record, where appropriate, disbursements between colleagues.

c) Plan the effective operation of the practice.
And in particular to:

    i.   Anticipate needs of colleagues and staff.

    ii.   Anticipate and organize locum cover.

    iii.   Keep an appointments diary.

    iv.   Anticipate the development of interdisciplinary collaboration for patient care.

    v.   Construct a business plan.

    vi.   Construct, review, and evaluate a business and practice management plan.

d) Buy/hire and maintain the practice.
And in particular to:

    i.   Negotiate financial loans as appropriate.

    ii.   Buy furnishings and fittings.

    iii.   Inspect regularly the property, furnishings, and fittings.

    iv.   Arrange repairs and replacements.

    v.   Install telecommunication systems appropriate for all situations (e.g. private communication, booking system, and siting for emergency use).

    vi.   Comply with statutory local planning, health, and safety requirements.

    vii.   Provide and monitor cleaning and laundry.

    viii.   Provide and use professional stationery.

    ix.   Provide and regulate an adequate heating and cooling system.

    x.   Provide appropriate means and equipment for dealing with clinical emergencies.

    xi.   Install resuscitation equipment.

    xii.   Keep an accident/incident book.

    xiii.   Install and maintain fire extinguishers.

    xiv.   Comply with fire regulations.

e) Keep appropriate case-history records.

And in particular to:
  i. Record name, address, date of birth, name of GP, health details, present medication, family and occupational details, case history, and details of examination and treatment for each visit.
  ii. Provide adequate storage and retrieval systems for relevant patient documentation.
  iii. Maintain up-to-date records.
  iv. Write in scientific language with accepted terminology.
  v. Record all findings, including negative findings.
  vi. Keep records securely, including confidentiality and compliance with data-protection act.
  vii. Treat records confidentially.

f) Recruit and manage staff.
And in particular to:
  i. Devise a person specification and a job description with performance standards and a contract in accordance with employment law and employees' rights.
  ii. Use appropriate recruitment strategies including adverts and selection interviews.
  iii. Plan and provide an induction and training plan for new staff.
  iv. Supervise and appraise performance regularly.
  v. Establish a grievance procedure.

A check-list is given below for further guidance:

In constructing a job description and performance review consider which of the following should be included:
  i. Arrangements for dealing with patients in confidence.
  ii. Limitations of authority and responsibility.
  iii. Making, rearranging, cancelling appointments.
  iv. Dealing with late arrivals, non-arrivals, late cancellations.
  v. Maintenance and updating of files in a confidential manner.
  vi. The system of keeping the practitioner informed of developments.
  vii. Clear definition of responsibilities, e.g. maintenance of property, cleaning, laundry, supplies.
  viii. Answering enquiries about suitability for treatment.
  ix. Criteria for dealing with a request for a domiciliary visit.
  x. Criteria for dealing with difficult patients.
  xi. Criteria for assessing a patient's immediate needs (e.g. help to go upstairs).
  xii. Clear guidance for obtaining feedback from patients (e.g. how they heard of the practice).
  xiii. Clear guidance for giving health-related information to the patient, face-to-face and by phone.

   xiv. How to approach other health professionals.

   xv. Clear indications of the style for correspondence.

   xvi. Information about the fee structure and a clear system for dealing with cash and cheques in payment of fees.

   xvii. Use of machines and equipment.

   xviii. Salary and other incentives and when they are to be reviewed.

g) Communicate outside the practice with health professionals/organizations/insurance companies.
   And in particular to:

   i. Keep in any easily retrievable form useful names, addresses and contact numbers, for example:

- colleagues in the practice
- other therapists
- medical practitioners
- paramedical practitioners
- health organisations
- health insurance companies
- next of kin
- employers of patients where necessary
- lawyers
- police
- local authority services.

   ii. Keep up to date with documentation on medico-legal requirements.

   iii. Keep up to date with changes in private health-insurance policy and inform the patient of his/her private health-insurance status.

h) Provide reports concerning patients for relevant agencies.
   And in particular to:

   i. Conform with patient consent requirements as appropriate.

   ii. Use appropriate phraseology and terminology.

   iii. Keep to deadlines.

   iv. Comply with any legal requirements.

Notes

Introduction

1. Personal communication to medical students following iatrogenic tragedy, *c.*1930, in *Medical Quotes*, eds. J. Daintith and A. Isaacs (Market House Books, Oxford, 1989).
2. D. M. Eisenberg *et al.*, 'Unconventional medicine in the United States: prevalence, costs and patterns of use', *N. Eng. J. Med.*, 328 (1993), 246–52.

Chapter 1

1. E. and P. Anderson, 'General practitioners and alternative medicine', *JRCGP*, 37 (1987), 52–5.
2. R. H. Bannerman *et al.*, *Traditional Medicine and Health Care Coverage* (World Health Organization, Geneva, 1983).

Chapter 2

1. Council of Europe, *Legislative and Administrative Regulations on the Use by Licensed Health Service Personnel of Non-Conventional Methods of Diagnosis and Treatment of Illness* (Council of the European Communities, Brussels, 1984).
2. G. J. Visser and C. Peters, 'Alternative medicine and general practitioners in the Netherlands: towards acceptance and integration', *Family Practice*, 7:3 (1990), 227–32.
3. Written question 1864/85, Madam Ursula Schleicher to Commission of the European Communities.
4. *Hansard*, vol. 518 (82), Col. 1,431 (1990).
5. Petition No. 359/87, Commission of the European Communities.
6. Written Question 1676/86, Mrs Beattie Webber (87/C149/33); Written Question 2303/88, Mr Derek Prague to Commission of the European Communities.
7. Written Question 762/90, Mr David Bowe to the Commission of the European Communities.
8. Written Question 2686/87, Andrea Fourcans to Commission of the European Communities.

9. Written Question 2962/86, Mrs Maij-Weggen to Commission of the European Communities.

10. EEC Directive 65/65.

11. T. Richards, 'Vitamins face control worldwide', *BMJ*, 305 (1992), 491.

12. European Commission, *Report of the Working Group on Dietary Supplements and Health Foods. Diet Integrators: A Discussion Paper 111/3767/91* (EC, Brussels, 1992).

13. A. Rogers, 'Europe: Homoeopathic Medicine', *Lancet*, 340 (1992), 167–8.

14. Written Question 1091/90, Mr Jean-Pierre Raffarin. The Official Journal of the EC C325, 24 Dec. 1990, p.30.

15. See n. 12 above.

16. See n. 2 above.

17. Research Council for Complementary Medicine, *Unconventional Medicine: An International Collaborative Research Project*. COST Project B4 (RCCM, London, 1992).

18. A. Abbott, 'Europe tightens rules that govern homoeopathic products', *Nature*, 359 (1992), 469.

Chapter 3

1. S. Fulder, *Handbook of Complementary Medicine*, 2nd edn. (Coronet, London, 1988).

2. British Holistic Medical Association, *A Response to the Government's Green Paper 'The Health of the Nation'* (BHMA, London, 1991).

3. S. J. Fulder and R. C. Munro, 'Complementary medicine in the UK: patients, practitioners and consultations', *Lancet*, 2 (1985), 542–5.

4. K. J. Thomas *et al.*, 'Use of non-orthodox and conventional health care in Great Britain', *BMJ*, 302 (1991), 207–10.

5. Consumers Association, 'Report on Regulation' (unpublished, 1992).

6. J. Ritchie *et al.*, *Access to Primary Healthcare: Report of the Office of Population Censuses and Surveys (OPCS) Social Survey Division* (HMSO, London, 1981).

7. See n. 2 above.

8. See n. 4 above.

9. J. M. D. Swayne, 'Survey of the use of homoeopathic medicine in the UK health system', *JRCGP*, 39 (1989), 503–6.

10. Office of Population Censuses and Surveys, *General Household Survey 1989*, Series GHS, No. 20 (HMSO, London, 1991).

11. See n. 4 above.

12. See n. 8 above.

13. This assertion may not hold true for all therapies; one recent survey (Medicare, 1991, unpublished) of over 1,000 randomly selected patients attending osteopaths suggested a broad social mix of patient work-load. Manipulative therapies may be in higher demand even among manual

workers. More evidence is needed in the form of reliable research from a broad range of therapies to establish the patient profile for non-conventional therapies.

14. See n. 4 above.
15. See n. 3 above.
16. See n. 2 above.
17. See n. 4 above.
18. See n. 8 above.
19. See n. 4 above.
20. See n. 3 above.
21. J. Murray and S. Shepherd, 'Alternative or additional medicine? A new dilemma for doctors', *JRCP*, 38 (1988), 511–14.
22. R. Wharton and G. Lewith, 'Complementary medicine and the general practitioner', *BMJ*, 292 (1986), 1,498–500.
23. D. T. Reilly, 'Young doctors' views on alternative medicine', *BMJ*, 287, (1983), 337–9.
24. D. T. Reilly and M. A. Taylor, *Developing Integrated Medicine: Report of the Research Council for Complementary Medicine (RCCM) Research Fellowship in Complementary Medicine 1987–90* (University of Glasgow, Glasgow, 1990).
25. General Medical Services Committee, *Your Choices for the Future: Results of the General Medical Services Committee Survey* (Electoral Reform Society, London, 1992).
26. *Doctor*, 16 July 1992.
27. E. and P. Anderson, 'General practitioners and alternative medicine, *JRCGP* 37, (1987), 52–5.

Chapter 4

1. R. Wharton and G. Lewith, 'Complementary medicine and the general practitioner', *BMJ*, 292 (1986), 1,498–500.
2. E. and P. Anderson, 'General practitioners and alternative medicine', *JRCGP*, 37 (1987), 52–5.
3. D. T. Reilly, 'Young doctors' views on alternative medicine', *BMJ*, 287 (1983), 337–9.
4. General Medical Council, *Professional Conduct and Discipline: Fitness to Practise* (GMC, London, Jan. 1969), 11.
5. British Medical Association, *Medical Ethics Today: Its Practice and Philosophy* (Professional & Scientific Publications (PSP), London, 1993).
6. M. Heseltine, *The Early History of the General Medical Council (1858–1886)* (The Medical Press, London, 1949).
7. S. Fulder, *Handbook of Complementary Medicine*, 2nd edn. (Oxford University Press, Oxford, 1988).
8. Royal College of Nursing, *Handbook 1992* (RCN, London, 1992).

9. British Medical Association, *Philosophy and Practice of Medical Ethics* (BMA, London, 1988).

10. Faculty of Homoeopathy Act (1950), 14 Geo. VI, c.20.

11. J. M. D. Swayne, 'Survey of the use of homoeopathic medicine in the UK health system', *JRCGP*, 39 (1989), 503–6.

12. J. Chisholm (ed.), *Making Sense of the New Contract* (Radcliffe Medical Press, Oxford, 1990).

13. Department of Health, *Statutory Instrument No. 635. The NHS (General Medical Services) Regulations 1992* (HMSO, London, 1992).

14. Royal College of General Practitioners, *Counselling in General Practice* (RCGP, London, 1992).

15. P. Pietroni, 'Beyond the boundaries: relationship between general practice and complementary medicine', *BMJ*, 305 (1992), 564–6.

16. British Medical Association, *Rights and Responsibilities of Doctors*, 2nd ed. (BMJ Publishing, London, 1992).

17. J. Murray and S. Shepherd, 'Alternative or additional medicine? A new dilemma for the doctor', *JRCP*, 38 (1988), 511–14.

18. King Edward's Hospital Fund for London, *Working Party on Osteopathy Report* (Kings Fund, London, 1991).

19. See n. 3 above.

20. D. T. Reilly and M. A. Taylor, *Developing Integrated Medicine: Report of the Research Council for Complementary Medicine (RCCM) Research Fellowship in Complementary Medicine 1987–90* (University of Glasgow, Glasgow, 1990).

21. T. Smith, 'Alternative medicine', *BMJ*, 287 (1983), 307–8.

22. Gallup Poll for the British Chiropractic Association (Jan. 1990, unpublished).

23. C. Budd *et al.*, 'A model of cooperation between complementary and allopathic medicine in a primary care setting', *BJGP*, 40 (1990), 376–8.

24. See n. 5 above.

25. P. Reason *et al.*, 'Towards a clinical framework for collaboration between general and complementary practitioners: discussion paper', *Jour. R. Soc. Med.*, 85 (1992), 161–3.

26. See n. 20 above.

27. 'Oxygen restriction and retinopathy of prematurity' (editorial), *Lancet*, 339 (1992), 961–3.

28. MRC Working Party, 'Medical Research Council European trial of chorion villus sampling', *Lancet*, 337 (1991), 1,491–9.

29. RCCM, 10th Anniversary Report 1983–1993 (RCCM, London, 1993).

30. A. M. Lilienfeld, 'Ceteris paribus: the evolution of the clinical trial', *Bull. Hist. Med.*, 56 (1982), 1–18.

31. A full discussion of the ethical problems in conducting clinical trials, particularly the difficulties in obtaining informed consent, is given in the BMA publication on medical ethics, n. 5 above.

32. M. Peckham, 'Research and development for the NHS', *Lancet*, 338 (1991), 367–71.

33. A. F. Long and T. A. Sheldon, 'Enhancing the effectiveness and accuracy of purchaser and provider decisions: overview and methods', *Quality in Health Care*, 1 (1992), 74–6.

34. Research Council for Complementary Medicine, *Tenth Anniversary Report* (RCCM, London, 1992).

35. House of Lords Select Committee on Science and Technology, *Priorities in Medical Research* (HMSO, London, 1988).

36. R. D. Tonkin, 'Role of research in the rapprochement between conventional medicine and complementary therapies: discussion paper', *Jour. R. Soc. Med*, 80 (1991), 361–3.

37. See e.g. R. Smith, 'Where is the wisdom?' *BMJ*, 303 (1991), 798–99.

38. P. Fisher *et al.*, 'Complementary medicine', 299 (1989), 1,401–2.

39. See n. 20 above.

40. V. S. G. Murray, 'Investigating alternative medicines', *BMJ*, 304 (1991), 11.

41. See n. 29 above.

Chapter 5

1. P. Pietroni, 'Beyond the boundaries: relationship between general practice and complementary medicine', *BMJ*, 305 (1992), 564–6.

2. *Hansard*, vol. 489, col. 1,379–416 (HMSO, London, 1987).

3. BMA, *Memorandum on the Theory, Technique and Practice of Osteopathy* (BMA, London, 1935).

4. See e.g. G. Larkin, 'Orthodox and osteopathic medicine in the inter-war years', in M. Saks (ed.), *Alternative Medicine in Britain* (Clarendon Press, Oxford, 1992).

5. *Hansard*, vol. 518, no. 82, col. 1,431–2 (HMSO, London, 1990).

Chapter 6

1. Consumers Association, 'Report on regulation' (unpublished, 1992; update).

2. S. Fulder, *Handbook of Complementary Medicine*, 2nd edn. (Oxford University Press, Oxford, 1988); R. Thomas (ed.), *1990 Natural Medicine Practitioners' Yearbook* (Journal of Alternative and Complementary Medicine, Tunbridge Wells, 1991).

Chapter 7

1. P. Vaughan, *Doctors' Commons: A Short History of the British Medical Association* (Heinemann, London, 1959).

2. Training Agency, *Development of Assessable Standards for National Certification. Guidance Note 2: Developing Standards by Reference to Functions* (Department of Employment, London, 1989).

3. Consumers Association, *Regulation of Practitioners of Non-Conventional Medicine* (Consumers Association, London, 1992).

4. T. W. Meade *et al.*, 'Low back pain of mechanical origin: randomised comparison of chiropractic and hospital outpatient treatment', *BMJ*, 300 (1990), 1,431–7.

5. E. Davenas *et al.*, 'Human basophil degranulation triggered by very dilute antiserum against IgE', *Nature*, 333 (1988), 816–18.

6. (Editorial), 'When to believe the unbelievable', Ibid.

7. J. Maddox *et al.*, '"High-Dilution" experiments a delusion', *Nature*, 334 (1988), 287–90.

8. J. Kleijnen *et al.*, 'Clinical trials of homeopathy', *BMJ*, 302 (1991), 316–23.

9. See e.g. C. A. Vincent and P. H. Richardson, 'The evaluation of therapeutic acupuncture; concepts and methods', *Pain*, 24, 1–13.

10. Clement-Jones *et al.*, 'Increased beta-endorphin but not met-enkephalin levels in human cerebrospinal fluid after acupuncture for recurrent pain', *Lancet*, 2 (1980), 946–9.

11. D. Larrey *et al.*, 'Hepatitis after germander (*Teucrium chamaedrys*) administration: another instance of herbal medicine hepatotoxicity', *Ann. Intern. Med.* (1992), 117, 129–32.

12. J. H. Galloway *et al.*, 'Potentially hazardous compound in a herbal slimming remedy', *Lancet*, 340 (1992), 179.

13. See e.g. R. S. MacDonald and C. M. J. Bell (1990), 'An open controlled assessment of osteopathic manipulation in nonspecific low-back pain', *Spine*, 15 (1990), 364–70.

14. C. Patel *et al.*, 'Controlled trial of biofeedback-aided behaviourial methods in reducing mild hypertension', *BMJ*, 282 (1981), 2,005–8.

Index

OXFORD

MORE OXFORD PAPERBACKS

This book is just one of nearly 1000 Oxford Paperbacks currently in print. If you would like details of other Oxford Paperbacks, including titles in the World's Classics, Oxford Reference, Oxford Books, OPUS, Past Masters, Oxford Authors, and Oxford Shakespeare series, please write to:

UK and Europe: Oxford Paperbacks Publicity Manager, Arts and Reference Publicity Department, Oxford University Press, Walton Street, Oxford OX2 6DP.

Customers in UK and Europe will find Oxford Paperbacks available in all good bookshops. But in case of difficulty please send orders to the Cash-with-Order Department, Oxford University Press Distribution Services, Saxon Way West, Corby, Northants NN18 9ES. Tel: 0536 741519; Fax: 0536 746337. Please send a cheque for the total cost of the books, plus £1.75 postage and packing for orders under £20; £2.75 for orders over £20. Customers outside the UK should add 10% of the cost of the books for postage and packing.

USA: Oxford Paperbacks Marketing Manager, Oxford University Press, Inc., 200 Madison Avenue, New York, N.Y. 10016.

Canada: Trade Department, Oxford University Press, 70 Wynford Drive, Don Mills, Ontario M3C 1J9.

Australia: Trade Marketing Manager, Oxford University Press, G.P.O. Box 2784Y, Melbourne 3001, Victoria.

South Africa: Oxford University Press, P.O. Box 1141, Cape Town 8000.

MEDICINE IN OXFORD PAPERBACKS

Oxford Paperbacks offers an increasing list of medical studies and reference books of interest to the specialist and general reader alike, including The Facts series, authoritative and practical guides to a wide range of common diseases and conditions.

CONCISE MEDICAL DICTIONARY
Third Edition

Written without the use of unnecessary technical jargon, this illustrated medical dictionary will be welcomed as a home reference, as well as an indispensible aid for all those working in the medical profession.

Nearly 10,000 important terms and concepts are explained, including all the major medical and surgical specialities, such as gynaecology and obstetrics, paediatrics, dermatology, neurology, cardiology, and tropical medicine. This third edition contains much new material on pre-natal diagnosis, infertility treatment, nuclear medicine, community health, and immunology. Terms relating to advances in molecular biology and genetic engineering have been added, and recently developed drugs in clinical use are included. A feature of the dictionary is its unusually full coverage of the fields of community health, psychology, and psychiatry.

Each entry contains a straightforward definition, followed by a more detailed description, while an extensive crossreference system provides the reader with a comprehensive view of a particular subject.

Also in Oxford Paperbacks:

Drugs and Medicine   Roderick Cawson and Roy Spector
Travellers' Health: How to Stay Healthy Abroad 2/e
Richard Dawood
I'm a Health Freak Too!
Aidan Macfarlane and Ann McPherson
Problem Drinking   Nick Heather and Ian Robertson

SCIENCE IN OXFORD PAPERBACKS

Oxford Paperbacks' expanding science and mathematics list offers a range of books across the scientific spectrum by men and women at the forefront of their fields, including Richard Dawkins, Martin Gardner, James Lovelock, Raymond Smullyan, and Nobel Prize winners Peter Medawar and Gerald Edelman.

THE SELFISH GENE

Second Edition

Richard Dawkins

Our genes made us. We animals exist for their preservation and are nothing more than their throwaway survival machines. The world of the selfish gene is one of savage competition, ruthless exploitation, and deceit. But what of the acts of apparent altruism found in nature—the bees who commit suicide when they sting to protect the hive, or the birds who risk their lives to warn the flock of an approaching hawk? Do they contravene the fundamental law of gene selfishness? By no means: Dawkins shows that the selfish gene is also the subtle gene. And he holds out the hope that our species—alone on earth—has the power to rebel against the designs of the selfish gene. This book is a call to arms. It is both manual and manifesto, and it grips like a thriller.

The Selfish Gene, Richard Dawkins's brilliant first book and still his most famous, is an international bestseller in thirteen languages. For this greatly expanded edition, endnotes have been added, giving fascinating reflections on the original text, and there are two major new chapters.

'learned, witty, and very well written . . . exhilaratingly good.' Sir Peter Medawar, *Spectator*

'Who should read this book? Everyone interested in the universe and their place in it.' Jeffrey R. Baylis, *Animal Behaviour*

'the sort of popular science writing that makes the reader feel like a genius' *New York Times*

Also in Oxford Paperbacks:

The Extended Phenotype   Richard Dawkins
The Ages of Gaia   James Lovelock
The Unheeded Cry   Bernard E. Rollin

SCIENCE IN OXFORD PAPERBACKS

Oxford Paperbacks offers a challenging and controversial list of science and mathematics books, ranging from theories of evolution to analyses of the latest micro-technology, from studies of the nervous system to advice on teenage health.

THE AGES OF GAIA
A Biography of Our Living Earth
James Lovelock

In his first book, *Gaia: A New Look at Life on Earth* (OPB, 1982), James Lovelock proposed a startling new theory of life. Previously it was accepted that plants and animals evolve on, but are distinct from, an inanimate planet. Gaia maintained that the Earth, its rocks, oceans, and atmosphere, and all living things are part of one great organism, evolving over the vast span of geological time. Much scientific work has since confirmed Lovelock's ideas.

In this new book, Lovelock elaborates the basis of a new and unified view of the earth and life sciences, discussing recent scientific developments in detail: the greenhouse effect, acid rain, the depletion of the ozone layer and the effects of ultraviolet radiation, the emission of CFCs, and nuclear power. He demonstrates the geophysical interaction of atmosphere, oceans, climate, and the Earth's crust, regulated comfortably for life by living organisms using the energy of the sun.

'Open the cover and bathe in great draughts of air that excitingly argue the case that "the earth is alive".' David Bellamy, *Observer*

'Lovelock deserves to be described as a genius.' *New Scientist*

'He is to science what Gandhi was to politics.' Fred Pearce, *New Scientist*

Also in Oxford Paperbacks:

What is Ecology? Denis Owen
The Selfish Gene 2/e Richard Dawkins
The Sacred Beetle and Other Great Essays in Science
Chosen and introduced by Martin Gardner

OXFORD LIVES

Biography at its best—this popular series offers authoritative accounts of the lives of famous men and women from the arts and sciences, politics and exploration.

'SUBTLE IS THE LORD'

The Science and the Life of Albert Einstein

Abraham Pais

Abraham Pais, an award-winning physicist who knew Einstein personally during the last nine years of his life, presents a guide to the life and the thought of the most famous scientist of our century. Using previously unpublished papers and personal recollections from their years of acquaintance, the narrative illuminates the man through his work with both liveliness and precision, making this *the* authoritative scientific biography of Einstein.

'The definitive life of Einstein.'
Brian Pippard, *Times Literary Supplement*

'By far the most important study of both the man and the scientist.' Paul Davies, *New Scientist*

'An outstanding biography of Albert Einstein that one finds oneself reading with sheer pleasure.' *Physics Today*

Also in the Oxford Lives series:

Peter Fleming: A Biography   Duff Hart-Davies
Gustav Holst: A Biography   Imogen Holst
T. H. White   Sylvia Townsend Warner
Joyce Cary: Gentleman Rider   Alan Bishop

RECREATIONS IN MATHEMATICS

Recreations in Mathematics covers all aspects of this diverse, ancient, and popular subject. There are books on puzzles and games, original studies of particular topics, translations, and reprints of classical works. Offering new versions of old problems and old versions of problems thought to be new, the series will interest lovers of mathematics—students and teachers, amateurs and professionals, young and old.

THE PUZZLING WORLD OF POLYHEDRAL DISSECTIONS
Stewart T. Coffin

This fascinating and fully illustrated book examines the history, geometry, and practical construction of three-dimensional puzzles. Containing solid puzzles, such as burrs, Tangrams, polyominoes, and those using rhombic dodecahedron and truncated octahedron, this collection includes a variety of unsolved and previously unpublished problems.

MATHEMATICAL BYWAYS IN AYLING, BEELING, AND CEILING
Hugh ApSimon

Set in the fictional villages of Ayling, Beeling, and Ceiling, and requiring little formal mathematical experience, this entertaining collection of problems develop a wide range of problem-solving techniques, which can then be used to tackle the more complex extensions to each puzzle.

Also available:

The Mathematics of Games   John D. Beasley
The Ins and Outs of Peg Solitaire   John D. Beasley